EVEN THE
STIFFEST
PEOPLE
CAN DO THE
SPLITS

EVEN THE STIFFEST PEOPLE CAN DO THE SPLITS

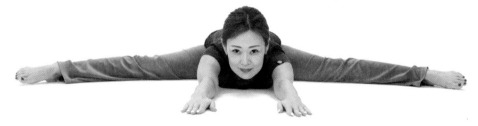

A 4-WEEK STRETCHING PLAN TO ACHIEVE AMAZING HEALTH

EIKO

RODALE
wellness

Live happy. Be healthy. Get inspired.

Sign up today to get exclusive access to our authors, exclusive bonuses,
and the most authoritative, useful, and cutting-edge information on health, wellness,
fitness, and living your life to the fullest.

Visit us online at RodaleWellness.com
Join us at RodaleWellness.com/Join

Copyright © 2017, 2016 by Eiko

Originally published in Japan with the title DONNANI KARADA GA KATAIHITODEMO BETTATO KAIKYAKU DEKIRUYONINARU SUGOI HOHO by Sunmark Publishing, Inc., Tokyo, Japan in 2016.

English translation rights arranged with Sunmark Publishing, Inc., through InterRights, Inc., Tokyo, Japan and Gudovitz & Company Literary Agency, New York, USA.

The proverbs and sidebars on pages 43, 51, 57, 77, 83, 93, 103, 105, and 121 were added by Rodale for this edition.

Rodale books may be purchased for business or promotional use or for special sales. For information, please e-mail: BookMarketing@Rodale.com.

Printed in the United States of America
Rodale Inc. makes every effort to use acid-free ⊗, recycled paper ♲.

Book design by Amy C. King and Jan Derevjanik

Library of Congress Cataloging-in-Publication Data is on file with the publisher.
ISBN 978-1-63565-178-2

Distributed to the trade by Macmillan
2   4   6   8   10   9   7   5   3   1   hardcover

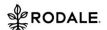

RODALE.

Follow us @RodaleBooks on

We inspire health, healing, happiness, and love in the world.
Starting with you.

There is nothing that cannot be achieved with firm determination.

–JAPANESE PROVERB

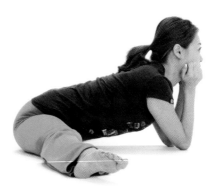

Table of Contents

ACT TWO: SHORT STORY

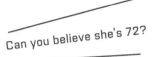

Can you believe she's 72?

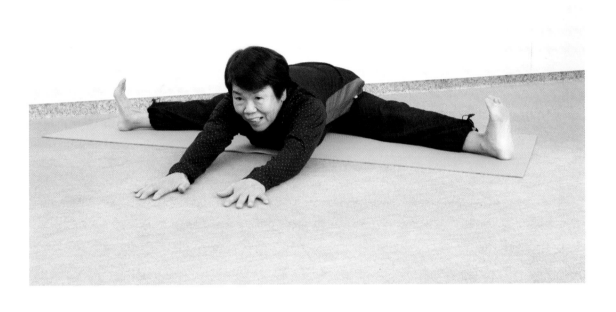

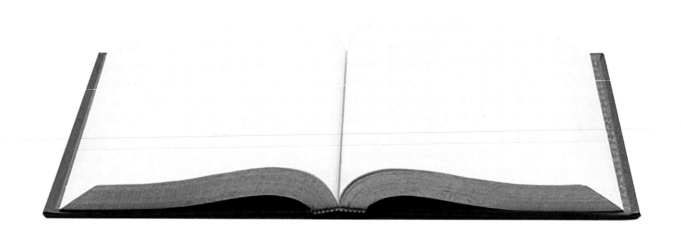

After some practice, you can be flat
like this book.

When I was in my twenties, I worked as an aerobics instructor. Over time my interests shifted to yoga and I decided to try to become a yoga instructor. There was one thing that bothered me back then, though: I wasn't very flexible. I suffered from backaches, and yoga movements were difficult for someone as inflexible as I was. Most of all, though, I wasn't much of an example for my students. I mean, if I were looking for a yoga teacher, I certainly wouldn't choose someone who wasn't flexible. That's when I launched a plan to remake my body.

Being able to do a pancake split, where you bring your upper body down flat to the floor while doing a middle split, is a symbol of having a flexible body. At the time, I could spread my legs out pretty well but I didn't have the flexibility to bring my upper body down to the floor. So I started doing research to identify what stretches I needed to do in order to be able to achieve the pancake. As long as I was at it, I wanted to develop a method that was reproducible—one that other people who struggled with flexibility could use, too. I tried all sorts of things day after day. The method I came up with proved really popular among my students. Before long, those who had said they were so inflexible they

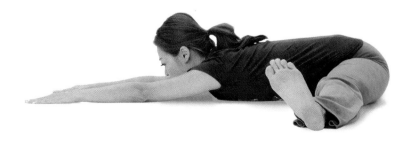

were embarrassed to come to yoga class were talking instead about how their newfound flexibility had changed their lives.

People in the media found out and I started getting offers to promote my method with a video. I was completely shocked when the video I made describing my method for the splits was viewed more than 6 million times. Who knew so many people wanted to be able to do the splits?

And now I've been given the opportunity to put out this book. What a surprise! After all, it's unheard of to have a whole book dedicated just to doing the splits. When the editor Seiichi Kurokawa made a special trip down from Tokyo to see me, I couldn't help but ask if he was sure he could really make a book out of my method.

But if we were going to make a book, I wanted it to be a good one. I wanted people who may have developed an inferiority complex because they were inflexible as kids to savor the sense of joy and exhilaration that comes with being able to do the splits. I wanted them to experience how smooth their everyday movements could become.

While making this book, I further improved my method for learning the splits so that now it's possible to achieve the pancake split in only about four weeks. By following the Splits in Four Weeks program, which I'll be introducing shortly, even people who have been inflexible since they were children and people whose bodies have

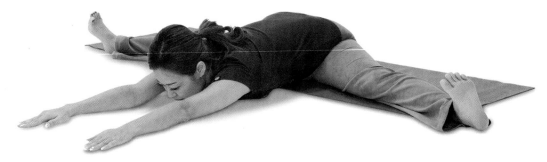

stiffened up as they've gotten older ought to be able to do the splits. The program changes a little bit each week so you can stick to it without getting bored. Being able to really feel a difference should also boost motivation.

After the Splits in Four Weeks program, the book includes a short story called "How Are You Going to Achieve Anything If You Can't Even Do the Splits?" It's a heartwarming story about Makoto Oba, who has had low flexibility ever since he was a child, and his colleague, Ai Umemoto, who has been looking for a new challenge to break out of a rut. They team up to try to achieve the pancake splits in a short time by putting my Queen of Splits method to the test. Who could have imagined the splits as the topic of a short story? This, too, might be something unheard of. The story's characters and settings are fictitious, but the Splits in Four Weeks program they follow and the other advice it contains are all things I hope you'll put into practice. Don't skip it, because it has all sorts of valuable hints. The four-week program shown on pages 12 to 33 is shown again within the pages of the short story, broken down week by week for easy reference.

The story is very realistic because it was written based on the experiences of people who have actually tried the Splits in Four Weeks program—what was a struggle, what was troubling, and what felt good. I'm sure reading it will boost your motivation.

Sure, it's only the splits. But it's so much more than the splits.

When you sweep away your inflexibility complex, you're going to want to congratulate yourself. The confidence that comes from "getting over it" is sure to suddenly make the rest of your life a little brighter. Please experience for yourself how refreshing it feels to do the splits.

Okay, let's get started.

Eiko, the Queen of Splits

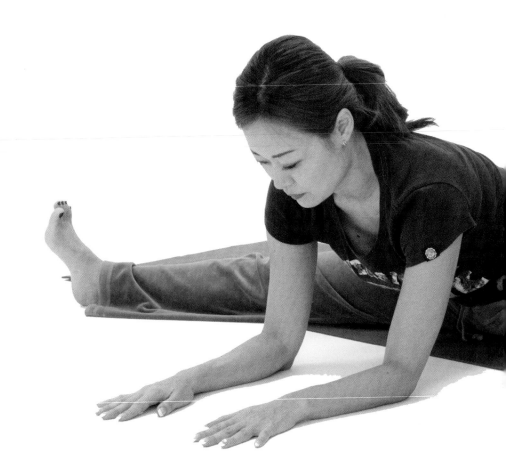

How
This
Book
Defines
the
Splits

* If you can put both of your elbows on the floor, you've done it!

* If you spread your legs wide while keeping your knees straight, lean your upper body forward, and touch the floor with both elbows, you've achieved the splits.

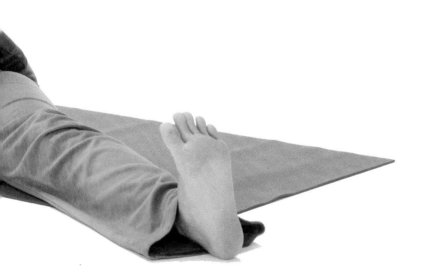

SUGAKO NISHINO
(72)

I started going to Eiko's studio at the age of 70. At first I couldn't spread my legs at all but I practiced what I had been taught every day while watching television and after about two months I surprised myself by being able to do a split. My body felt lighter and more mobile and I could run up the stairs to the third floor of my house without even getting winded. My waist tightened up and I was able to wear pants that I couldn't fit into before. Now I'm more limber than my 53-year-old daughter!

You Can Do the Splits at Any Age!

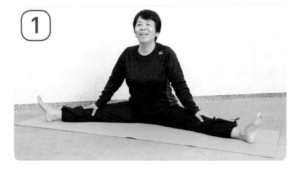

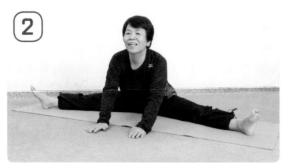

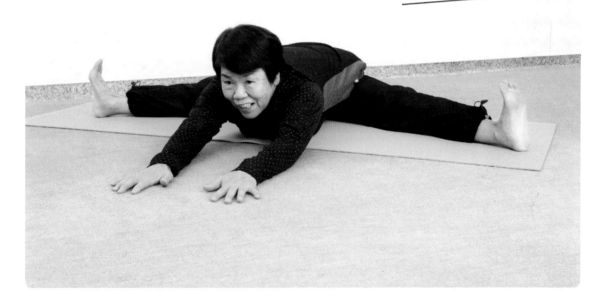

My waist got
thinner, too!

KEIKO ICHIKO
(68)

I was 63 when I first started going to Eiko's studio. Until then I couldn't lean forward at all when my legs were spread, but now I can bring my upper body down flat to the floor. My friends are all amazed. I even lost 11 pounds, and although I used to go to the hospital regularly for back pain, now it hardly bothers me at all. My knee joints used to hurt but they're much better now, and I can go up and down stairs without any trouble.

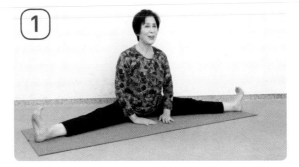

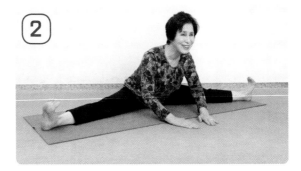

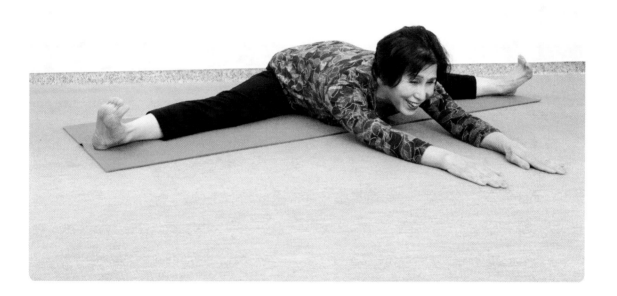

③

I lost 11 pounds and
no longer get backaches!

AKEMI HIRAOKA
(66)

I've been going to lessons once a week since I was 60. Everyone in my family is inflexible, but thanks to Eiko I've managed to become limber enough to do a pancake split. I can really feel the difference in my circulation. I used to have to wear socks to bed and pile on the blankets or else my feet would be so cold I couldn't sleep, but now I feel much warmer and sleep comfortably with fewer blankets. I'm really grateful for what Eiko taught me.

You Can Do the Splits at Any Age!

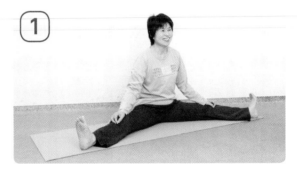

1

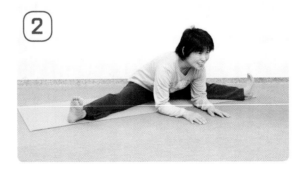

2

My circulation has improved
and I feel much warmer.

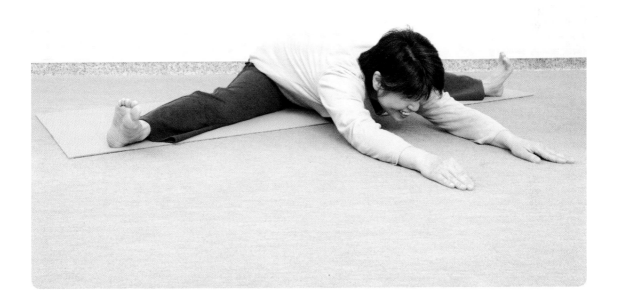

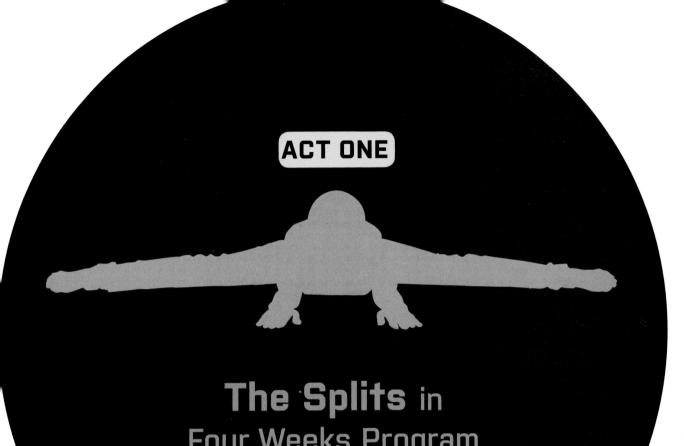

ACT ONE

The Splits in
Four Weeks Program
to Help Even Inflexible People
Achieve Perfect Splits

The time for perfect splits has finally arrived!

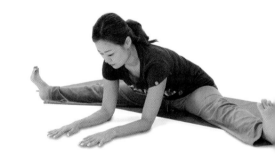

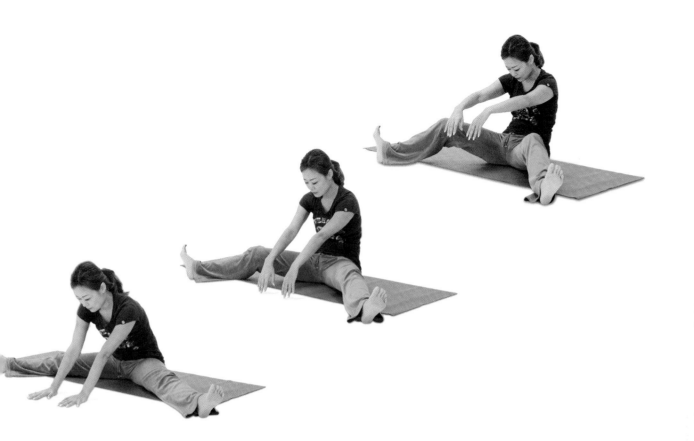

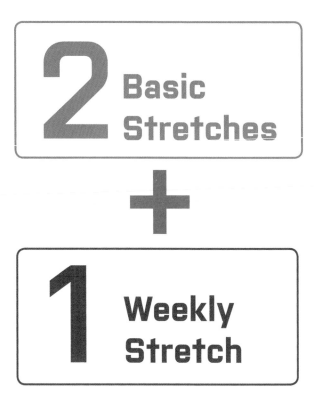

For the next four weeks, you'll do three types of stretches each day. The first two are basic stretches that you'll do every day until you achieve the splits. The third is a weekly stretch that changes as you advance each week.

BASIC STRETCHES

1 Towel Stretch

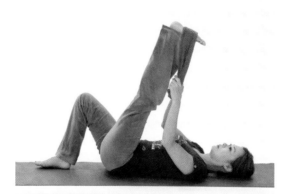

2 Sumo Stretch

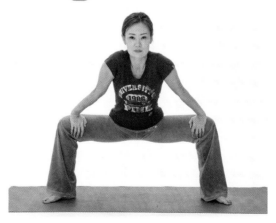

WEEKLY STRETCHES

Week 1 Inner Thigh Stretch

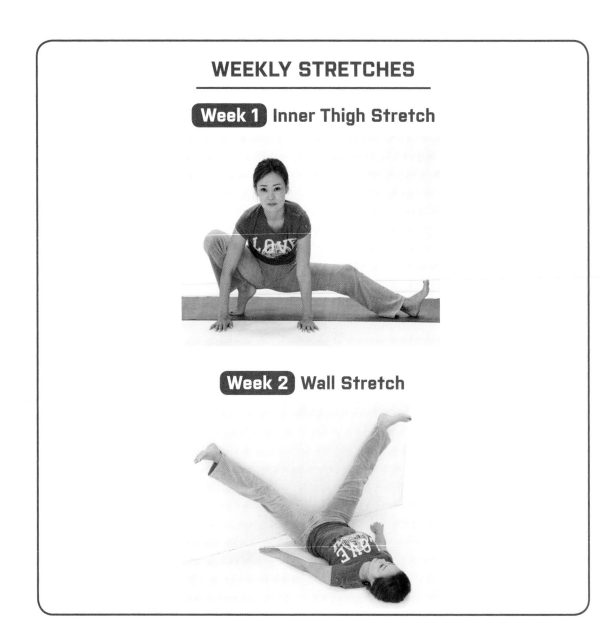

Week 2 Wall Stretch

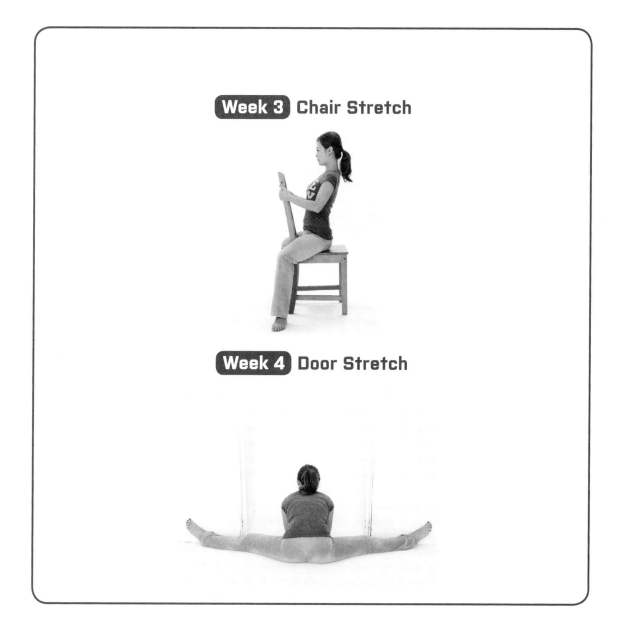

Week 3 Chair Stretch

Week 4 Door Stretch

BASIC STRETCHES TO DO EVERY DAY FOR FOUR WEEKS

There are two basic stretches: the towel stretch and the sumo stretch. The key is to stretch only so far that it hurts in a good way. Be careful not to overdo it when starting out.

1 Towel Stretch

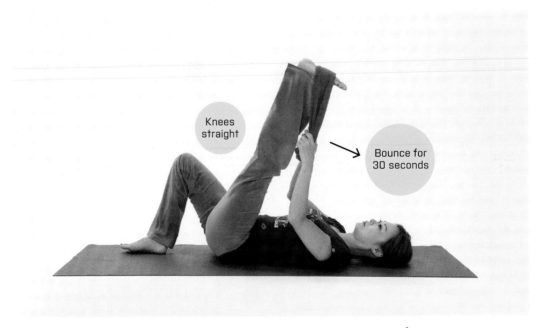

Knees straight

Bounce for 30 seconds

Loop a hand towel over the underside of one foot, extend your leg (keeping your knee straight) and pull the towel toward your head with both hands, bouncing for 30 seconds. Do the same with the other leg.

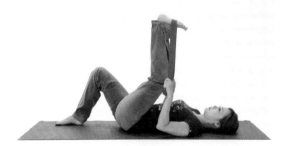

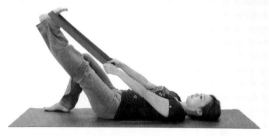

If you bend your knee, you won't get much of a stretch. If this stretch is difficult, use something longer, like a bath towel, rope, or belt.

If this stretch is difficult, it's okay not to draw your leg closer. Just be sure to keep your knee straight.

2 Sumo Stretch

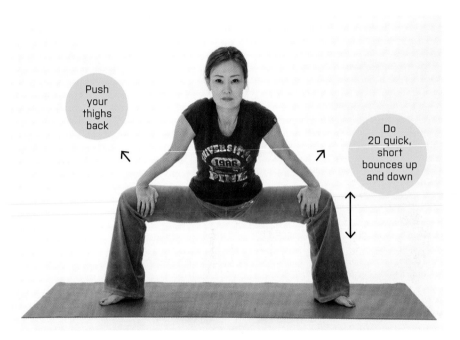

Push your thighs back

Do 20 quick, short bounces up and down

1 Point your knees outward, spread your legs about twice the width of your shoulders, lower your backside, and place your hands on your inner thighs near your knees. Your thighs should be parallel to the floor.

2 Bounce up and down in quick, short movements, about 20 times.

3 Next, stretch the groin and back by twisting each shoulder toward the middle in turn while pushing harder with your hands.

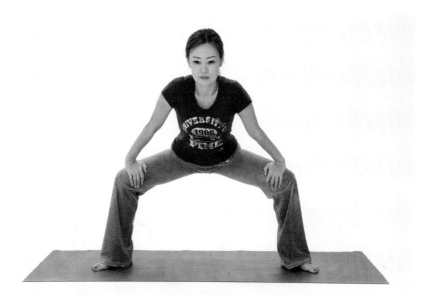

This is
is
OK

If this stretch is difficult, it's okay not to lower your hips all the way.

WEEK

1

Inner Thigh Stretch

In addition to the two basic stretches, you'll do one stretch that changes each week. For the first week, this is an inner thigh stretch. After you've finished each day's routine, be sure to try doing the splits.

1 Towel Stretch

2 Sumo Stretch

+

3 Inner Thigh Stretch

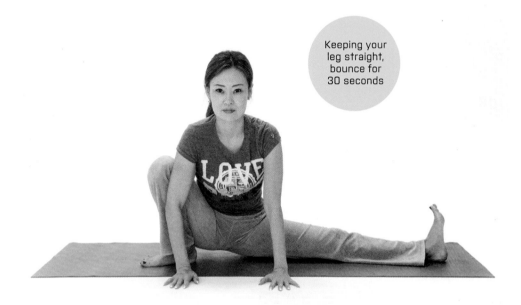

Keeping your leg straight, bounce for 30 seconds

With one knee bent, stretch out the other leg to the side, bouncing for 30 seconds. Do the same with the other leg.

**Don't
Do
This**

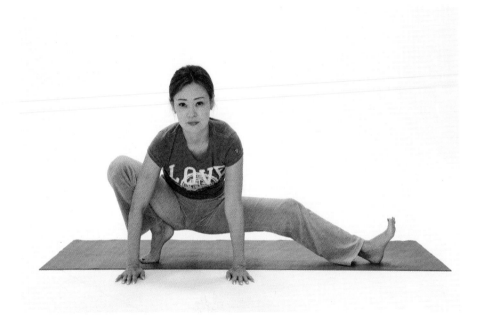

This stretch won't be effective if
both of your knees are bent.

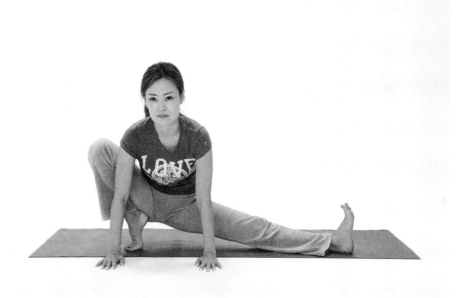

If you're inflexible, it's okay if the heel
of the bent leg leaves the floor.

When you're done with week one, try doing the splits to check your progress!

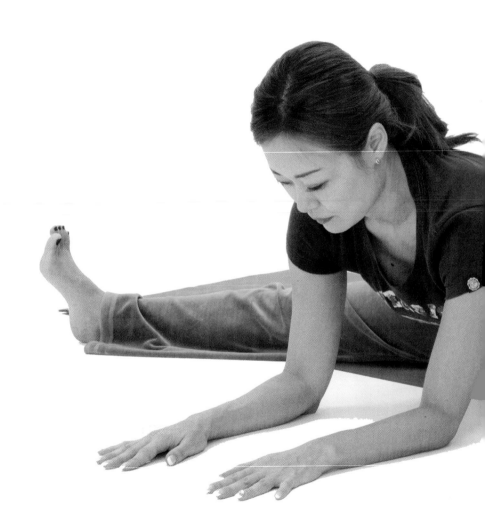

Sit with your legs spread out as far as they will go without bending your knees and lean your upper body forward. Your ultimate goal is for both elbows to touch the floor. Having someone photograph you each day from the same position is an easy way to track your progress. (You can also try taking pictures of yourself in a mirror.)

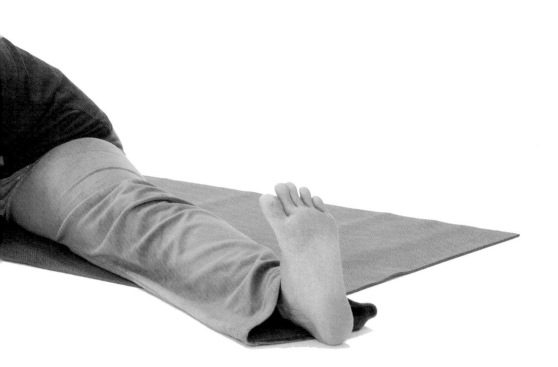

WEEK

2

Wall Stretch

The weekly stretch for week two uses a wall to bring you closer to the splits. Since the wall supports the weight of your legs, you can increase the intensity without bending your knees and without pushing too far.

BASIC STRETCHES TO DO EVERY DAY

1 Towel Stretch

2 Sumo Stretch

3 Wall Stretch

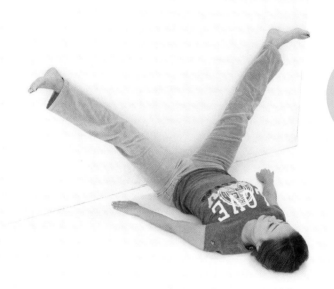

Stretch for 1 to 2 minutes while bouncing

1 Position your backside along the wall, extend your legs toward the ceiling, then open up your legs.

2 Place your legs against the wall, spread them as far as you can without bending your knees or pushing too far, and stretch for 1 to 2 minutes while bouncing your legs apart.

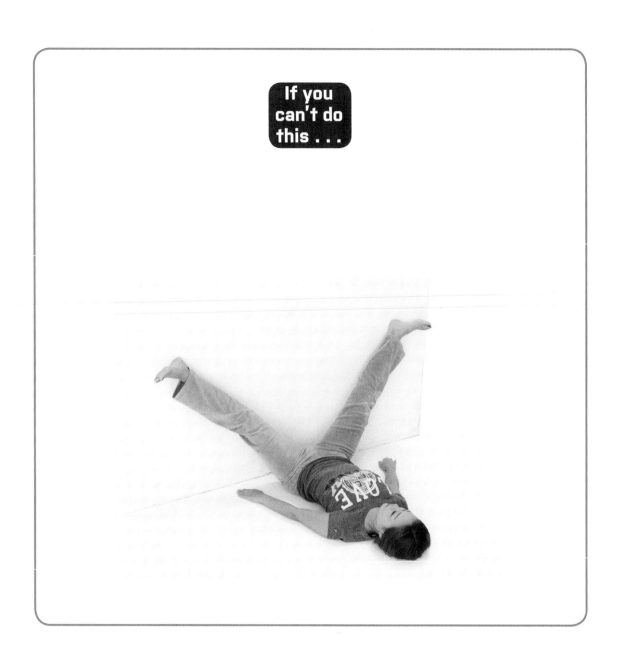

This is OK

Adjust the intensity of the stretch by varying how open your legs are and the distance between your backside and the wall. If this stretch is difficult, it's okay to only go as far as you can.

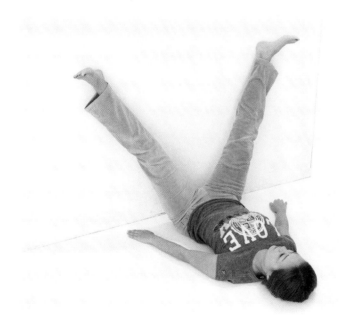

When you're done with week two, try doing the splits to check your progress!

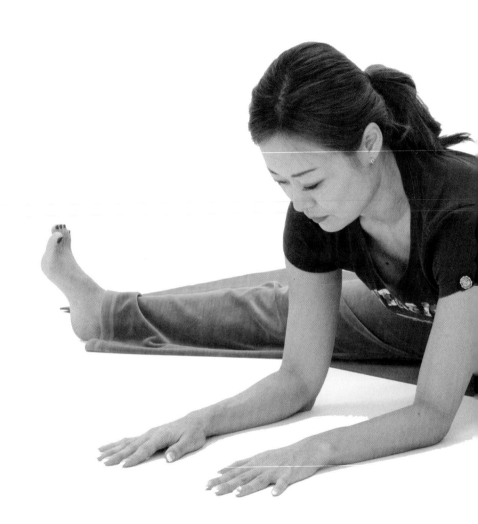

Sit with your legs spread out as far as they will go without bending your knees and lean your upper body forward. Your ultimate goal is for both elbows to touch the floor. Having someone photograph you each day from the same position is an easy way to track your progress. (You can also try taking pictures of yourself in a mirror.)

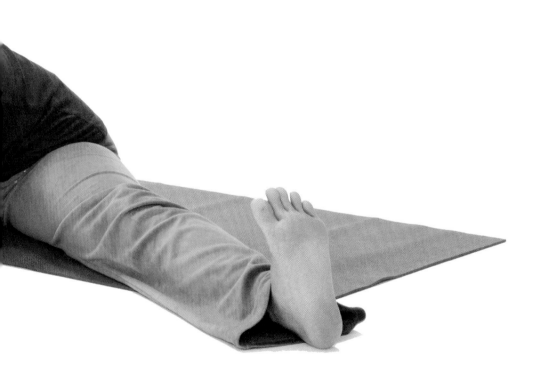

WEEK

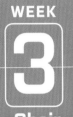

3

Chair Stretch

For week three, you'll do a chair stretch, which applies pressure to your hip joints. The key is that the back of the chair enables you to freely adjust the intensity.

BASIC STRETCHES TO DO EVERY DAY

1 Towel Stretch

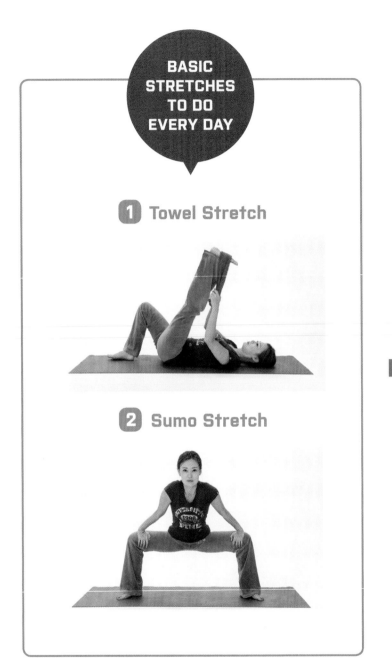

2 Sumo Stretch

+

24

3 Chair Stretch

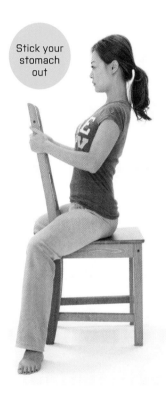

Stick your stomach out

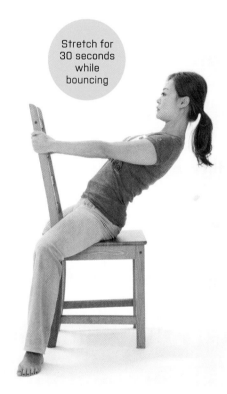

Stretch for 30 seconds while bouncing

1 Straddle the chair facing the seat back with your feet in line with the back of the chair. Grabbing the seat back with both hands, stick your stomach out.

2 Lean your upper body back while pulling on the seat back, open up your knees, and stretch your hips for 30 seconds while bouncing.

When
you're
done with
week
three,
try doing
the splits
to check
your
progress!

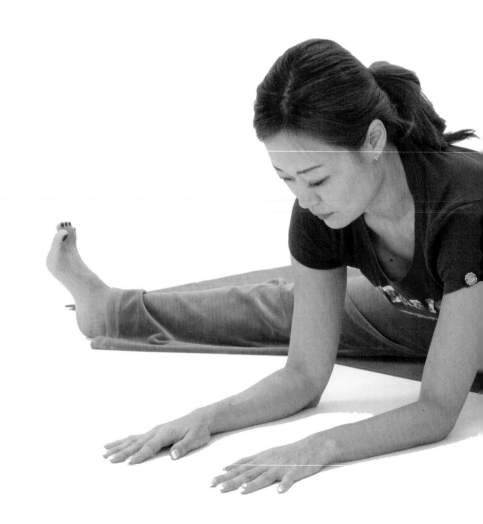

Sit with your legs spread out as far as they will go without bending your knees and lean your upper body forward. Your ultimate goal is for both elbows to touch the floor. Having someone photograph you each day from the same position is an easy way to track your progress. (You can also try taking pictures of yourself in a mirror.)

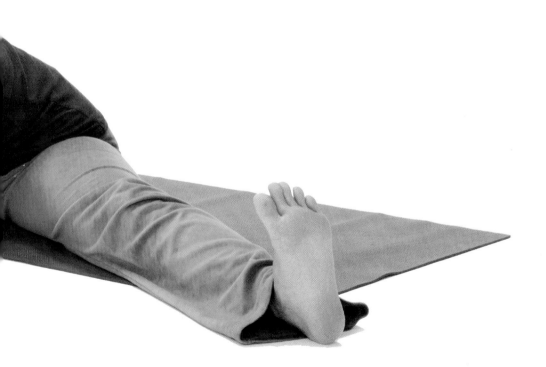

27

WEEK

4

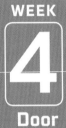

Door Stretch

Finally, the last week! With the door stretch, since you let the walls take care of your legs, your goal of the splits should seem closer than ever. If you don't have a door to use, try the frog stretch.

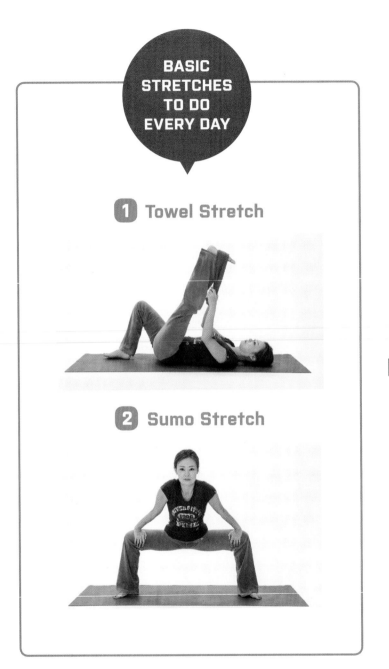

BASIC STRETCHES TO DO EVERY DAY

1 Towel Stretch

2 Sumo Stretch

+

3 Door Stretch

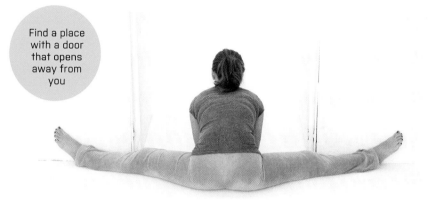

Find a place with a door that opens away from you

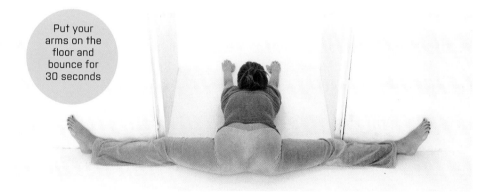

Put your arms on the floor and bounce for 30 seconds

1 Find a doorway whose walls on both sides are in the same plane and whose door opens away from you, then sit down in front of it with your legs spread.

2 Supporting your outstretched legs with the walls, lower your upper body forward and place your arms on the floor, stretching for 30 seconds while bouncing.

If you don't have a door:

FROG STRETCH

Spread your legs wide with your
toes pointing out. Lower your hands
to the floor and support your upper
body, which will want to tumble forward, stretching for 30 seconds. If
you cannot reach the floor with your
hands, support your upper body by
resting your elbows on your thighs
near your knees.

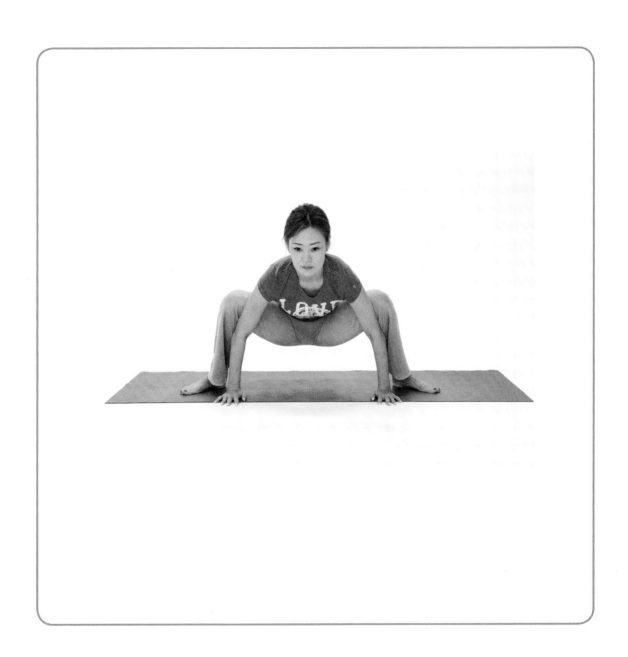

After four weeks, you're sure to see a change.

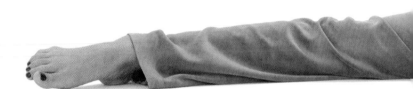

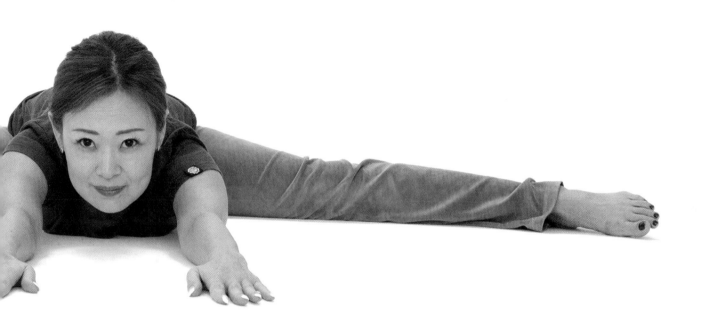

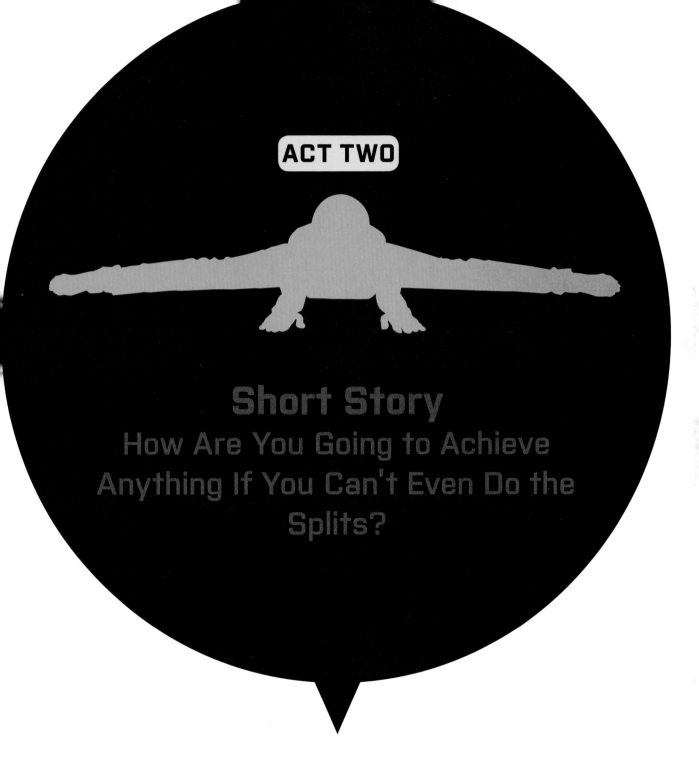

ACT TWO

Short Story
How Are You Going to Achieve
Anything If You Can't Even Do the
Splits?

CAST OF CHARACTERS

Makoto Oba
(40 years old)

↓

Sales manager at a trading company. Lives with his wife and his son, Tsubasa, a soccer-mad second grader. Once a competent soccer player, he now has a textbook "dad bod." Recently, he has started to feel anxious about getting old. He has a gentle personality and modest achievements at work.

Ai Umemoto
(32 years old)

↓

A career-track employee in Oba's department. Unable to give herself over completely to her job, her days feel less than ideal and low on self-actualization. Now in her thirties, she finds it harder to stay slim, tougher to stick to a diet, and can feel her body stiffening up. She is single and looking for love.

Tetsuya Hori
(45 years old)

↓

Recognized by all as the star of the company's middle ranks. Graduated from the same university as Oba a few years earlier. After single-handedly reviving the moribund Osaka office during a solo posting there, he has now returned to headquarters as a departmental director. He carries himself elegantly and has a cheery, positive outlook. Is adept at motivating and charming subordinates. His secret has an unlikely source!

Eiko
(50 years old)

↓

Yoga instructor based in Osaka. Her video on how to do the splits, describing a method based on her own experience as someone who was once inflexible and not only couldn't do the splits but even hurt herself, became a huge viral hit with millions of views. She taught Hori to do the splits in just four weeks while he was posted to Osaka.

Prologue 1

MAKOTO OBA'S SUNDAY

"Dad, come on! You promised!"

Sandwiched between piles of documents and struggling to put together materials for his presentation, Makoto Oba saw Tsubasa suddenly appear before him, dribbling a soccer ball. Although his son was proud of his brand-new uniform, it had been bought with room to grow and the baggy clothes seemed to wear the boy.

Oba knew his son liked to play soccer, but wasn't it dangerous to be kicking the ball around in the apartment? And if he was wearing his uniform, why hadn't he gone to practice with the youth team he was so excited to be a member of? Oba was suddenly overcome by a wave of drowsiness and both Tsubasa's uniform and his computer screen faded off into the distance. *Sorry, son. Dad needs a little sleep. It may not look it but I'm really busy. Please, I just need a few more . . .* Oba pleaded in his head as he rolled over sluggishly on the bed.

"Shoot!"

Seeing a golden opportunity, Tsubasa kicked a well-aimed shot that caught his father right in the lower back, finally rousing him from his dreams. *That's right! I was supposed to play soccer with Tsubasa!*

Tsubasa went to soccer practice every Sunday morning, usually not coming home until sunset. This week, though, the third-graders and the other older teammates he played with were off for a day of training elsewhere and the younger kids had the day off. Tsubasa wasn't happy about this, so Oba had promised to help him with his training today, something he hadn't done in a while.

The clock showed it was already 9 a.m. His wife had probably already headed off to the apartment-complex community meeting. Tsubasa had watched all his morning TV shows and was ready to go. Oba had been at his computer until 3 a.m. getting ready for his Monday presentation, trying not to carry the work over into today so he could keep his promise to Tsubasa.

Oba was surprised, given how rudely he'd been awakened, how good it felt to be up and how light his body felt. Now that he was 40, his work at the office was more difficult and not particularly glamorous, while the talented youngsters who had come on board during the hiring slump were developing fast. Whether because of the pressure or his age, he almost always felt some measure of pain and fatigue in his shoulders, back, lower back, or hip joints. Today, though, he felt refreshed: one of those too-good-to-be-true days that came maybe once a month.

"All right, Tsubasa," Oba said as he kicked off the covers. "Hold on just a minute and I'll get ready to go."

Instead of making lame excuses and moving at a snail's pace as usual, today he was going to give Tsubasa his full attention. The lightness in his body wasn't the only reason he was in a good mood: tomorrow, he knew, an old mentor he looked up to would be coming back to the office.

Oba quickly washed his face, shaved, and started to pull on his socks. Recently, he had begun to feel how his body was tightening up. It was getting harder to pull up his socks without leaning his body forward. It used to be enough just to crouch down when tying the laces of his running shoes, but now he always plopped himself down onto the step at the entrance. He tried to pass this off as a matter of maintaining a dignity appropriate to his age, but the fact was that it was just hard to do without sitting down. His "dad belly" was starting to show, too.

Oba had been a soccer-crazy boy himself once. Inspired by the *Captain Tsubasa* comic book, he had raced around the playing field from elementary school through junior high and never been relegated to being a sub. He gave up the sport in high school because of the long commute, but then joined a serious soccer club at university that often held matches with outside teams. That's where he met his wife.

Even after starting work and getting married, and up until Tsubasa was born, he had been an active member of a soccer team made up of graduates of his school. In the last few years, though, as he grew busy with work, fell out of shape, and started to gain weight, his role had been limited to keeping things rolling at team get-togethers and end-of-the-year parties.

Although he wished he could follow the example of the older members of the team who still ran around with energy even in their fifties, he didn't do anything about it but sigh.

It was a gorgeous day. As they waited for an elevator in the outside corridor, Mt. Fuji looked beautiful in the distance. It would probably be a few years before Tsubasa was able to notice such beauty on his own.

Oba was secretly pleased that Tsubasa had taken to soccer so completely. Four years ago he had stretched to buy their current apartment in the hope that his son would come to enjoy the sport. Soccer was popular in the area, which was not only home to a J-League professional team but also had many fields in an expansive riverside park less than ten minutes away on foot. There was even a soccer school run by by a former J-Leaguer.

Tsubasa had made a lot of friends through soccer, and the area really seemed to have become his hometown. The monthly mortgage payments were a heavy burden, but Oba was happy they had made the move. Even though he did have a tendency to overestimate his son's talents, Oba had no illusions that Tsubasa would grow up to become a professional soccer player. Still, if that were something he wanted to pursue, it was certainly better to start early. After all, according to one theory he had heard, the nervous system was fully formed by the age of 10.

With as good as I feel today, I just might still have it in me. Instead of letting my boy have all the fun, maybe I ought to get back into soc-cer. With such thoughts running through his mind for the first time is a long while, Oba regarded his pudgy reflection in the elevator's mirror.

That morning, the soccer fields along the river were nearly empty, perhaps because all the older kids were off elsewhere. They could put together whatever kind of training menu they pleased. Tsubasa was juggling a ball, anxious to get moving.

They decided to start off with a game where Tsubasa would dribble toward the goal and Oba would try to steal the ball from him. As he often reminded his son, playing one-on-one was the cornerstone of soccer practice.

It had been about six months since Oba had done a proper workout with Tsubasa—maybe even longer—and he was taken by surprise. Once just a little squirt running around in circles, Tsubasa had made impressive progress. He was now better able to dodge Oba's attacks and had gained a lot of speed.

Having planned to go easy on his son, Oba quickly had to readjust. He wasn't going to be much of a training partner unless he really gave it his all. As a parent, though, this unexpected turn of events made him very happy. The time had finally arrived when they could enjoy soccer together, and he found himself thrilled beyond his imagining.

At the same time, the sensation from back when he had played soccer gradually started to return to him: how to step, how to handle his upper body, when to move in close to his opponent, the *thwack* of the ball, the pleasant feeling of reading his opponent and attacking at the limits of his speed and technique.

Tsubasa, you've gotten so good! And look at me. I've still got it, don't I?

Oba's feeling of elation, however, was short-lived. Even though his mind was reacting, his body was unable to translate its directives into play. He quickly grew fatigued. Out of breath. Soon he couldn't keep up with Tsubasa any longer. Unwilling to admit defeat, he took a long stride and at that moment he missed his footing and—his momentum carrying him forward—took a magnificent spill.

"Dad, are you all right?"

Tsubasa peered down at him, looking concerned. Oba felt something odd in his mouth that made it hard to speak, and his knee, which he seemed to have landed on, throbbed in pain. Although he didn't seem to have sprained an ankle or torn an Achilles tendon, he couldn't be sure whether he had instinctively tucked and rolled or just been lucky to land without serious injury.

Oba staggered to his feet. Trying to at least sound tough, he said, "I'm all right. Why don't you practice by yourself a bit?" and left the playing field, testing his body for damage as he went.

Totally pathetic. I can't believe how poorly I move!

Oba realized immediately that it had been a mistake to start playing right away without doing a proper warm-up, especially since he exercised so infrequently.

He couldn't lie to himself, though. The reality was that he was clearly aging, that his body was no longer as limber as it once was and had stiffened up. He didn't yet feel old in his mind, but his body was no longer able to carry out the instructions his brain was still convinced it could execute.

DOING THE SPLITS KEEPS YOU YOUNG!

Practicing the splits is great for your joint health,[1] flexibility, and balance—qualities that become more and more important as we age. All of these things factor into how much range of motion we retain, our physical independence, and overall quality of life. Balance is especially important, as falls are the leading cause of death from injury in elderly people, even healthy ones.[2]

Stretching exercises like the splits have even been proven to help with major health issues like Parkinson's[3] and cardiovascular disease[4] by encouraging muscle strength, motor control, and better circulation. See page 93 to learn how the splits can even prevent injuries.

In the end, his practice with Tsubasa ended up a mix of avoidance and nursing himself along, which came as a real shock to Oba. Back at home, he found himself unable to relax even after settling onto the couch. Was he really so past his prime, well on the way to becoming a feeble old man? Was this what everybody meant when they talked about getting old?

It hurt Oba deeply to know that his growing son had witnessed his humiliation.

The feeling was similar to the sadness he always felt when thinking about his younger, more capable colleagues at work. Oba's title marked him as a manager, but he had no direct subordinates. He was no longer confident that he was doing better work than they were.

A major personnel reshuffle was going to be officially announced at work the next day. An older colleague who had gone to the same university and helped him out a lot over the years would be returning to headquarters as his boss, taking over one of the most promising positions in the company after making an unqualified success out of a sink-or-swim situation at a branch office.

His old friend, though, was not the type to push his way to the top by kicking others out of the way, or so nakedly ambitious as to be unapproachable. Indeed, he was elegant, bright, vigorous, and charismatic—a man of character who held himself to high standards while bringing out the best in others.

At 45 years old, he still went out shopping with his daughter to fashionable places like Shibuya and Harajuku. *How is that even possible? How does he manage to be such a class act? What are the odds that I'll look like that in five years?* As he mulled over such thoughts in his head, Makoto Oba's Sunday drew to a close.

AI UMEMOTO'S SUNDAY

All of a sudden it was after seven at night.

The apartment in which Ai Umemoto lived alone was quiet and bare white. In order that it not seem too forlorn, she had left the television on with the volume down even though she had no interest in what was on.

It suddenly occurred to her that she hadn't spoken to anyone all day.

Tomorrow there would be a major organizational restructuring and shuffling of personnel at the trading company where she worked. Though it would not mean any major changes in her own job, the consolidation of her department would bring the arrival of a new boss.

The week was set to begin on Monday with a long all-hands meeting where team members would introduce themselves. Rather than conducting individual interviews, the new departmental director and the executive in charge wanted to make sure the team was all on the same page by getting everyone together and having each present a status report and describe their expectations going forward.

Umemoto compiled her results over the past two years—a general analysis of the fields with which she now worked, an analysis of the clients and prospective clients she currently handled and her thoughts on their future prospects, an update on the status of new projects, and her current progress in reaching the targets she had set for herself in the last company review—organizing all of this information in a format for easy presentation.

It would have been better for her to complete this task during working hours the previous week but, unable to clear her desk of routine work, she had ultimately ended up bringing it home with her over the weekend.

To tell the truth, she was in a heavy mood. One of her few remaining unmarried friends, someone with whom she really felt at ease, had invited her to lunch that day, but she had turned down the offer because she needed to finish her presentation. At the same time, it wasn't as if throwing away a precious holiday had resulted in a particularly productive day.

She was in a department at headquarters that was considered a desirable placement, her performance assessments were not bad, and her colleagues often complimented her on the way she applied herself to her work.

Umemoto herself was convinced that she was one of those people who were capable of doing good work, and took particular pride in her observational and analytical skills. She maintained, on the surface, a cheery disposition because she knew this gave her a clear advantage at work. And yet, as she was painfully aware, she could not deceive herself.

Was this all she had accomplished at work over the past two years? Surely she could have done more.

Wasn't she prone to skimp on preparations, and to squeak out of tight spots with stopgap excuses papered over with a smile? How much longer would she be able to rely on such improvisation and last-minute tricks when the competition was so tough inside and outside the company?

At the same time, she tended to slip into the bad habit of pretending to be busy. By focusing on the amount of time she spent on her work rather than its quality, she convinced herself she was working hard. Over time, the state of being busy brought, all by itself, its own modest, intoxicating pleasure. Ultimately, though, this was just an avenue of escape from a less-than-fulfilling personal life.

Feeling hungry, Umemoto tied up her disheveled hair, threw on a parka, slipped on a pair of sandals, and headed off to the neighborhood grocery to get some food. She knew that this was the hour when discount stickers were applied to the ready-to-eat foods at the deli counter, and that on a Sunday there would be fewer rivals than usual.

Along the way, no matter how hard she tried to shake them off, she could not keep the small regrets of the day from bubbling to the fore. If she was going to fritter away her time pretending to work even when she was at home with no one watching, it really would have been better to just go out to lunch with her friend.

Blaming everything on her work, she thought, so much remained undone: the trips she wished to take but hadn't, the diet she wanted to maintain but couldn't, the expensive yoga classes she never attended but continued to pay for. And yet it was not as if work offered a sense of fulfillment that made it all worth it. In the end, unable to stick with anything, she mastered nothing.

A head spinning with such thoughts left little room for forward progress. Umemoto realized she was in even worse shape than usual.

At 32 years old, she had been working for a decade, and had been with her current company for six years. Oddly, she had never been particularly offended when called a career woman. What she disliked was her own inability to fully become a career woman despite wanting to do so, and her irritation with herself for failing to apply herself completely to her work, instead doing things by half.

Umemoto found it impossible to organize her own work. Lacking confidence, she found it hard to take responsibility. In the end, she always waited for instructions, and although she was certainly able to tolerate working hard, she never really gained a true sense of accomplishment.

She was still unable to break out of the mold of a "cute, competent girl at the office." Something was missing, but her image of what that might be remained vague.

At the supermarket deli section, Umemoto found, as expected, a whole slew of items priced to move, marked with colorful "half off" stickers. Although the chilled air coming from the refrigerated cases was a bit depressing, she started to feel a little better.

She chose a salad topped with chicken, some simmered vegetables, and boiled fish. Given her gradually increasing weight, it would be best to refrain from carbohydrates at this hour. Since she wasn't exercising, she would have to find a way to make adjustments on the intake side.

She also purchased half a loaf of French bread and a cup of instant soup, but these were strictly for tomorrow's breakfast. She then picked up some beer, which she had run out of, and other items before paying for her purchases with a credit card that partnered with an airline. She started to wonder when she would ever be able to use the miles she was accumulating, which set her off on another descending spiral of negative thinking.

She had not had a partner since she broke up, at the age of 26, with the person she'd been dating since her student days. That was just after she had changed jobs and come to work at her current company, a time when she thought she was serious about trying to reach the next level. Back then she just hadn't been able to think about marriage.

One by one, her friends got married. Some returned to work after taking maternity or childcare leave, while others applied their skills to jobs they could do at home or dedicated themselves to homemaking. These friends certainly faced struggles of their own, but they all seemed to be facing married life and child rearing—all the major life changes—head on while enjoying themselves, too.

Umemoto's mother took little interest in her work. Indeed, even if she had wanted to be interested, the fact that she had lived as a housewife ever since her own marriage meant that she knew little of the working world, and reacted to Umemoto's stories with no more than a, "Well, that sounds hard."

At the same time, the pressure from her mother concerning marriage and children only grew more persistent with each passing year. She was always talking about how so-and-so in the neighborhood had just been blessed with her second child or how some cousin had just celebrated her wedding in Hawaii.

Whenever Umemoto checked Facebook or Instagram, she always found them overflowing with stories like that. Sometimes, looking through them all was just too distressing.

Did others her age share the same kinds of worries she felt? If they did, maybe they just never posted about them on social networking sites.

Umemoto understood why her mother worried about her. She wasn't feeling particularly anxious herself yet. She didn't want to think her chance for love had passed, and she did want to get married and have children if the opportunity presented itself. The fact was, though, that her days were exceedingly dull, passing in a present that kept repeating itself without ever revealing where it was leading.

Back at the apartment, Umemoto used the microwave to warm up the simmered vegetables and boiled fish she had bought, then looked through tomorrow's presentation one more time as she ate.

The overall flow was good, covering all the essential points, but the quality and quantity of the data that grounded her analysis of current conditions and outlook for the future was weak, leading to fuzzy conclusions. There was no time left, though, to obtain materials for a more careful analysis that would turn things around and strengthen her argument. She certainly couldn't start the new week by staying up all night.

She stared vacantly for a bit, decided to let time take its course, put aside the presentation, and went to bed. If her lack of preparation showed, she would just have to take the scolding she deserved.

Suddenly she felt like having a beer. The dinner she had bought for herself had not been nearly enough. She was still hungry. Abandoning her plans of just thirty minutes before, she ate the French bread meant for breakfast. Hearing herself make the excuse that she was eating in the proper order of vegetables, proteins, and then carbohydrates only made her feel wretched.

HOW CAN THE SPLITS
HELP YOUR DIET PLAN?

It may seem like a strange claim that practicing the splits can help you stick to your diet. But research has shown that exercises like stretching have been proven to enhance self-control, can help influence people to make better dietary decisions,[5] and can curb hunger.[6] Regular stretching can assist weight loss by encouraging better digestion.[7]

Taking a few mindful minutes to practice the splits before you eat a meal can also slow you down and make you more aware of your portions and eating habits. By relieving stress, you're also letting go of any emotions or tension that could have influenced your food choices in negative ways. Stretching also increases body awareness, making you cognizant of your body's positioning and strength. Over time, this awareness helps build self-confidence and self-love. Better weight management often naturally follows this healthy mind-set!

This was why she could never stick firmly to a diet. As for the 8:00-p.m. yoga class she had signed up for—partly as a reason to leave work at a reasonable hour—after attending a few sessions, she had stopped going and now found it difficult to start up again. Since reaching her thirties, she had found it harder to keep weight off, and could feel herself stiffening up. Exercise was more difficult than it used to be, and it was probably a bit late to take up tennis or running.

What was she doing? How could everything be so half-baked? Where was she headed? Umemoto let out a deep sigh.

Oba, who worked in the same department and had always been supportive of Umemoto at work, had told her that the new director coming in to run the department was an old mentor.

The conversation had left an impression on her because Oba, who ordinarily didn't talk about other people very much, had seemed ready to leap from his chair as he praised his old friend without reservation. At any rate, the new director was now the center of attention at work, having driven a magnificent turnaround in the sales team at the Osaka branch, which had been on the verge of being shut down. The rumors had even reached Umemoto, to whom he was a perfect stranger.

Oba said the new director, who had gone to the same university as he had, had taken him under his wing when he joined the company, had a gentle disposition, looked out for his juniors, was always stylish and well dressed, and was even devoted to his family, too. Did such supermen really exist?

Umemoto gave her presentation one final look, saved the changes, steeled herself, and then powered down her computer. And with this, Ai Umemoto's Sunday drew to a close.

THE SHOCK IN THE CONFERENCE ROOM

Sure enough, Umemoto's lack of preparation was duly noted at the company meeting, where it earned her a talking to.

Still, she didn't feel at all bad about it, especially compared to the way she had been going around in circles the night before. The new director, Tetsuya Hori, had given her the key points—and only the key points—that she needed to see things more clearly for herself, then provided suggestions for improvement and urged her to go through the presentation one more time, all the while maintaining a positive tone.

Recognizing that her new boss couldn't be fooled actually brightened Umemoto's mood. *All right,* she said to herself. *I'll redo it and get it right this time.* Oba didn't fail to note her renewed sense of resolve.

The meeting had started at one o'clock and gone on for nearly four hours, but from the opening remarks by the executive in charge and the new director through the individual presentations and discussion of shared objectives, Oba felt the time had been well spent. Indeed, the time had flown. He felt sure that everyone in the room saw in Hori an even more powerful presence than the one described in the rumors they had heard.

It wasn't just the content of the meeting, though, that impressed Oba so much. It was the way Hori handled himself so brilliantly, setting the scene, managing the meeting, keeping things entertaining, revealing his own feelings but also drawing out how everyone else felt. Most of Oba's interactions with Hori had been one-on-one, and though they had been friends for nearly 20 years, it had been a while since he'd seen his old friend in such a setting.

Oba was also a little anxious about his younger colleague Umemoto, who had been called out for her lack of preparation. She was amenable, cheerful, and a hard worker, but her work was rarely criticized and he wondered if it had come as a shock to her.

Most of all, he hoped she hadn't been left with a negative impression of Hori, the friend he thought so highly of. He was sure she would understand as she got to know him better, but he also wanted to be there for her on this first day under the new structure.

The department that Hori now led, the result of a consolidation, was a large one, with a staff of almost 50. Unless there was something really urgent, ordinary staff members would be unlikely to have the opportunity to speak with him casually in the course of their everyday work.

Oba checked in on Umemoto after the meeting. When their eyes met, she was the first to speak.

"Oba, you're friends with Director Hori, right? I'd like to talk to him in a little more detail about the things he pointed out in my presentation, but I'm not sure if I should just go up to him and ask directly. What do you think?"

If that's all Umemoto wanted, Oba was more than happy to help out. All he had to do was introduce her in the course of small talk to make sure that Hori would keep an eye on her going forward.

Unfortunately, it looked as if Hori was already caught up in a conversation with the executive who had been sitting beside him. Still in their seats, they had started to pull out papers. It looked like the beginning of a long conversation, so it seemed best not to interrupt. Meanwhile, all the other participants were leaving the room. It wouldn't do for just Oba and Umemoto to be left standing there alone.

"Let's wait outside until they're done," Oba said, ushering Umemoto into the hallway outside the conference room.

"Makoto, thanks. You're such a help! The new director went to the same university you did, right?"

"He was actually my recruiter when I was job hunting. I met him again at the new employee orientation and he's been a huge help to me ever since."

Umemoto could tell that Oba meant every word he said.

"He's amazing, isn't he?" said Umemoto. "Today's the first time I've seen him in action, of course, but just listening to him for a few hours made me think, you know, that he was the sort of person I could do anything for."

"Right," said Oba. "But the fact is, there's nothing we can do for him. I'm pretty sure we'll be relying on him."

Oba began explaining more about Hori's background. Two years ago there had been a plan to disband the sales team in Osaka—which had been performing particularly poorly at a time when company results were down overall. What could be sold off would be sold and everything else would be dealt with by traveling back and forth from headquarters. After a bit of confusion, it was decided that Hori would be sent in to run the place for three years, after which the branch would be shut down if things hadn't improved. There were, of course, some factional power dynamics at play, too.

Because his daughter had been facing school entrance exams, Hori left his family behind and went off to Osaka on his own. Nevertheless, he managed to turn things around there in just half the time allotted.

Apparently it only took a month before those who had looked coolly upon this sudden interloper from Tokyo instead regarded him with looks of respect. There were two things he said over and over again: "What are we working for?" and "I'll take responsibility." In this way he energized his subordinates and in just a year and a half managed to achieve results on a scale that left no room for complaint.

Hori had already been known as the ace of the company's middle ranks, but this feat put him a step or two ahead in the race for advancement. Today marked a triumphant return to Tokyo with a promotion to lead the newly consolidated headquarters sales team.

"But Oba, you must know a lot about what the new director's really like."

"Well, I suppose so. Can you believe he's forty-five?"

"He's certainly not your typical forty-five-year-old. He's not over-weight at all. He dresses well. And he carries himself with—I don't know—a certain elegance."

"Meanwhile, look at me with my potbelly. . . . But it isn't as if Hori's always been like that. In fact, I think it's something he's grown into over time, and especially during the last two years in Osaka. The two of used to go out for drinks when he came back to town and every time I saw him he seemed even more polished."

"I'm sure in no position to judge you for putting on a little weight, but how do you think he does it?"

"I wish I knew. I hear that since getting back to Tokyo, he goes out shopping with his daughter, who's in high school, and even runs more than three miles every morning with his son, who's in junior high."

Umemoto could feel herself becoming more relaxed. From the way Oba was talking, she could tell that the new director was someone she could trust, and with Oba smoothing the way, she was sure she would be able to build a good relationship with him. Given what an amazing person he seemed to be, she wanted to learn as much from him as she could, to steal all of his secrets, and she was fully committed to taking a positive approach.

The conference room door opened and the executive in charge walked out. Smiling, he looked back and said, "See you later, Hori. Keep it up." and shut the door behind him. Hori, however, did not come out.

"Hey," said Umemoto. "I wonder what happened to Director Hori?"

"When we left the room a minute ago it was just the two of them, right?"

Oba and Umemoto quietly put their ears to the door to see if they could get a sense of what might be going on inside, but they heard no voices or any other sounds. They looked at each other, and then Oba abruptly made as if to open the door.

"Wait!" Umemoto said. "Shouldn't you knock first?"

But before she could finish the sentence Oba had thrown open the door. The first thing that caught their eye was Hori with his jacket off, his legs spread out 180 degrees on the carpet of the conference room, and his upper body lowered to the floor.

HOW LOW CAN YOU GO?

(Explanation of the Amazing Forward Bend)

"Well, you've caught me in a compromising position, haven't you?" After momentarily looking flustered when he realized he'd been seen doing the splits, Hori immediately regained his composure with a sly joke. Even so, he did seem a little embarrassed.

Hori's attempt to deflect their attention, though, had no effect on Oba and Umemoto, who just stood there with their mouths open. There was just too much going on before their eyes to decide what to focus on first.

"I was just trying to reset after that long meeting," Hori said.

"Reset?" said Oba. "Why are you doing the splits? I've never seen anyone do the splits in person before!"

"Director Hori, you're so limber," said Umemoto. "But doing that on the carpet, won't your suit get dirty or torn?"

"I gained two things in Osaka," said Hori with a smile as he slowly stood up. "The first was the time I spent with my friends at the branch there and the things we accomplished together. The second was control over my body, which used to be really inflexible. Surprised you, didn't I?"

Hori adopted the same positive attitude as always, his expression radiant like the sun. Since Oba and Umemoto were still at a loss for words, he continued. "Can either of you do the splits?"

"Me?" said Oba. "Of course not. How about you, Umemoto?"

"Not me. I did try yoga for a while but I'm not very flexible and it didn't last long. You're amazing, Director Hori."

"Not really," he replied. "I used to be really stiff, too, but once I started trying, I was able to do the splits in about a month."

Oba and Umemoto couldn't believe it.

"Wait a minute, Tetsuya. You might have thought you were stiff, but you were actually a lot more flexible than most people, right?"

"Not really, Makoto. If I told you that just about anyone can learn to do the splits in a month—actually four weeks—just by doing some simple stretches, would you believe me? What about you—what was your name again?"

"Ai Umemoto. Um, frankly, I would find that hard to believe. It doesn't sound like something I could do."

"I don't know, Tetsuya," said Oba. "I've been feeling pretty stiff lately. It's getting harder to pull on my socks and shoes, and the other day I took a tumble while playing soccer with my son. Doing the splits sure seems like a long shot. Isn't it a matter of whether you're born flexible or not?"

Hori's expression took on a more determined look. "No, that's not it at all. Look, why not try it for yourself? Makoto, you know what a standing forward bend is, don't you?"

"Um, yeah. It's that thing chiropractors have you do where you bend forward and they say you're in good shape if you can touch the floor with your hands, right?"

"That's the one. I want the two of you to try it. Ai, you probably ought to slip off your pumps, first."

Following Hori's lead, Oba and Umemoto placed their materials on a desk, stood side by side, and began bending over at the waist.

"Keep your heels together with your toes slightly apart," said Hori. "That's right. Keep your knees straight. Don't bend them. And we're just taking a reading, here, so there's no need to push yourself too hard."

Neither Oba nor Umemoto reached anywhere near the floor. Even stretching out their fingers to the fullest they only made it as far as about halfway between the floor and their knees.

"This is hard," said Oba. "I can't do it at all."

"Okay, good," Hori said. "Both of you remember how far you reached."

"Um, Director Hori, is this supposed to get easier?"

Turning to Umemoto, whose doubts were written on her face, Hori pointed to the wall.

"The wall?" she asked.

"That's right. When the instructor I learned from showed me this stretch, I could feel my body start to loosen up all by itself."

A ONE-MINUTE STRETCH THAT WILL DRAMATICALLY IMPROVE YOUR FORWARD BEND

Stand in front of a wall. Pushing it with both arms extended, straighten your back leg to stretch your calf and Achilles tendon for 30 seconds. Then do the same with the other leg.

1. Be sure not to bend the knee of the leg you are stretching.

2. Keep the toes of both feet pointed straight at the wall.

3. Keep both heels flat on the floor.

4. There's no need to push the wall with all your might; just use your arms to support your body.

Doing as Hori indicated, Oba and Umemoto stretched each of their legs for 30 seconds in turn while pushing the wall.

"Okay," said Hori. "That's probably enough. Now try the forward bend again, like before."

When they did, the results were amazing. Both Oba and Umemoto could feel how they were able to bend farther forward than they had before. Their fingertips were so much closer to the floor that they could hardly contain themselves.

"Incredible," said Umemoto. "When I get to the point I reached before, it doesn't hurt at all this time."

"No kidding," said Oba. "What a shock. Who knew just one minute could make such a difference?"

"See?" said Hori. "When I first experienced this I was really surprised. I'd always been concerned about being inflexible, and then one day I ran across this video. . . ."

He stopped suddenly. "Hold on," he continued. "I'm supposed to be making the rounds to introduce myself. And you two must have had some reason for coming back."

"Tetsuya," said Oba. "Ai here has been thinking about what you said during the meeting and wanted some more advice before things got too busy, but then we were both so surprised to see you doing the splits . . ."

"That's right," Umemoto added. "The advice you gave me at the meeting really struck a chord, and seemed related to some things that have been worrying me. There were some things I wanted to ask, but then all of the sudden we were doing forward bends. . . ."

"I see," said Hori. "Sorry about that. You can ask me anything you want. Why don't we meet back here this evening to keep the conversation going?"

After they agreed to reconvene at seven thirty, Hori threw on his jacket and dashed from the room.

LIGHT THE FIRE OF THE SPLITS IN YOUR HEART

(Explanation of the Amazing Pair Stretch)

At seven thirty that evening, the three gathered again in the conference room. Hori brought a cold six-pack of beer and some snacks, though it was a mystery where he had found time in his busy day to buy them. Oba gave Hori some background on Umemoto's career to date and how she approached her work, and then Umemoto described her concerns and asked Hori for advice on how to overcome them.

Occasionally eliciting more information and sometimes offering encouragement, Hori provided sound advice to his subordinate, who was more than a decade younger than he was.

Seeing Umemoto's expression quickly brighten, Oba was both relieved and overcome with admiration. His old mentor really was something else. After this, Umemoto would be able to find her own way, and grow into her work, even if left to her own devices.

After the main topic had been addressed, Oba asked something he hadn't had a chance to that afternoon. "Tetsuya, why did being inflexible only start to bother you after moving to Osaka? I don't think you ever mentioned that before."

"Well," said Hori. "It's kind of personal. Something that had actually been on my mind for a long time."

"But Director Hori, you must have been really busy in Osaka," said Umemoto, asking a question that hit at the heart of the matter.

"Why choose a time like that to start learning to do the splits?"

"Two years ago," Hori began after a pause, "when I went to Osaka without my family, I felt a certain kind of pressure. Everybody's really happy with me now that the results are in, but back then I was more nervous than confident."

Oba found himself leaning forward and listening more attentively.

"I knew that if I was able to overcome that pressure," Hori continued, "I would come out on the other side a new, stronger me. I knew I also needed something other than work to anchor me, some kind of mental growth. And even though it may seem unexpected, for me that was the splits."

"That's what I don't understand, Tetsuya," said Oba. "Of all things, why the splits?"

Looking a bit bashful, Hori replied, "Like so many stories, it begins with a girl. A long time ago I really liked a girl on the gymnastics team. She carried herself so beautifully. Her grades were good and she had a real presence. I thought she was amazing. I was on the basketball team, so I always used to see her practicing in the gym. I'll never forget how casually and elegantly she seemed to do the splits when warming up. I wasn't limber at all and certainly couldn't to the splits, so she seemed awfully far away. At the time, I had a real inferiority complex about it."

"But Director Hori," Umemoto interrupted. "Didn't you ever tell her how you felt?"

"No," he replied. "I never said anything. I never even told my good friends that I liked her. It all seems pretty silly looking back now, but at the time I felt so strongly about her it just made her seem even further out of reach."

"But Tetsuya," said Oba, "if that was all there was to it, why is it any more than a bittersweet memory? Why decide to try to do the splits as an adult, and at the very moment you were embarking on such a sink-or-swim challenge in Osaka? I mean, you've already got a lovely wife and adorable kids, right?" This just didn't make sense to Oba.

"You're right, of course," said Hori, his expression starting to shift back into work mode. "Forget about the girl from gymnastics for a minute, and let me try to explain it as simply as possible. The way I saw at, it seemed like accepting that I wasn't able to do something was holding me back, giving me a reason not to outperform myself. I figured this was why I was so scared looking up at this huge wall in front of me—at the challenge of turning around the branch office in Osaka. Back in the day, she was so beautiful doing such smooth splits, and I was so uncool and inflexible—without ever realizing it, those feelings had been influencing my thinking and my way of looking at things, and all came flooding back at the moment I was faced with such a big challenge."

Hori's words seemed to resonate with Umemoto, who said, "I think I know what you mean."

"Sounds familiar?" said Hori. "Anyway, around that time I happened to learn about a video that was popular on the Internet called 'Stretches That Will Enable Even Inflexible People to Do the Splits.' At the time, it had been viewed more than a million times. This seemed like a happy coincidence and I watched it over and over. I thought that if I were able to learn to do the splits I might really be able to exceed my own limits, so I started to take stretching classes at the instructor's studio."

66

Oba had known Hori for nearly twenty years, but everything he was hearing today was completely new to him. "Still," he said, "you must have been more flexible then than we are now, right?"

"No," said Hori. "About the same, or maybe even worse."

"In that case, then," asked Umemoto, "when you decided to start stretching to do the splits, did you have a sense right away that you would be successful?"

"I never had any doubts," said Hori. "Much like the stretch we did for the standing forward bend earlier, when I did the first splits-related stretch my teacher taught me I was suddenly able to spread my legs surprisingly wide. Do you want to try it? But maybe you'd rather not sit on the floor. . . ."

"I know," said Oba. "We could get the picnic sheets we use for cherry-blossom viewing parties." He quickly went and got a few.

"All right, then," said Hori. "Makoto, you get to be the guinea pig. Your pants have a little leeway in them, right? Ai, you just watch for now."

Oba sat down on one of the picnic sheets.

"First," said Hori, "try doing a split cold. Just like this afternoon, we're going to start by checking how far you can go."

"No warm up or anything?" asked Oba. "This hurts. Trying to keep my knees from bending is really hard." Oba's legs were spread no more than maybe ninety degrees. Trying to spread them any farther made his knees bend.

"Okay," said Hori. "There's no reason to go beyond the point where it hurts in a good way. Now, maintaining the same position, how far you can lower your upper body toward the floor?"

Unfortunately, instead of Oba's body lowering toward the floor, it only leaned ever so slightly forward. He hurriedly dropped his hands to the floor.

"That's all right," said Hori. "Now we'll do another one-minute stretch. You'll be amazed at the difference it makes."

A ONE-MINUTE PAIR STRETCH THAT WILL SPREAD YOUR LEGS SURPRISINGLY WIDE

1 Form a facing pair of one person who will stretch and another who will provide support. The person doing the stretching spreads their legs as far as they will go and extends their arms forward. The supporter then slowly pulls their arms forward.

2 The person doing the stretching tries to lean back in the opposite direction from which their arms are being pulled. Do this for one minute.

Be careful not to bend your knees.

Hori gently pulled Oba's arms forward while Oba leaned his upper body back in the opposite direction.

Looking slightly worried, Umemoto asked, "Makoto, does it hurt?"

"No," he said. "My upper body's actually fine. You know, Tetsuya, this looks like it would stretch the upper body but it's actually stretching the backs of the legs, isn't it?"

"Oh, you catch on fast. You've got a knack for this."

After the one-minute stretch was over, Oba tried spreading his legs again. This time he was able to spread them much wider than he had just a few minutes before, and was able to lean his upper body forward, too!

"Wow," Oba said. "I never thought just one little stretch would make such a difference."

"Makoto," said Umemoto, "you sure look more limber than before!"

Looking pleased to see how excited the others were, Hori said, "That stretch is easiest to do with a partner, but there's a way to do it by yourself, too. I was alone in Osaka so I always did it by myself."

"So you used to do this every day at home, then?" Oba asked.

"That's right. When you're just getting started, it's especially important to keep it up every day. Right now, you're a lot looser than you were, but if you don't keep it up you'll go right back to being as tight as you were before. It's really important to keep stretching every day, especially at the beginning." Hori had the same expression as when he gave advice about work.

"But Director Hori," said Umemoto, "you didn't come up with this stretch yourself, did you?"

"Of course not," he said. "I learned it from Eiko, the teacher who posted the splits video I mentioned earlier."

"Wait," said Oba. "You mean you didn't just watch the video, you met her in person and learned from her directly?"

"That's right. I thought the program was a good fit, so I did some research and as luck would have it, Eiko turned out to be a yoga instructor in Osaka. I figured it had to be fate. Eiko offered yoga classes so I signed up right away. It was mostly women in the class, though, so I did feel a little out of place." Hori was smiling, but spoke as if this was a matter of course. He said he still practiced even now that he had returned to Tokyo, using Eiko's DVD as a guide.

Since Umemoto had taken yoga lessons, she thought she understood what Hori meant. "I took yoga classes once," she said, "so I can imagine you must have stood out."

"Well, yes. I was usually the only guy there. More than that, though, I really felt a lot in common with Eiko, who herself had once struggled with a lack of flexibility. It helped that she could understand my feelings of inferiority, and I was committed to staying interested in this new world I had stepped into, and focused on trying to get beyond the old me. It didn't bother me, really, and I even made some talkative new friends."

"So," said Oba, "you started out just like I am today and were really able to do the splits in just a month?"

"That's right," said Hori with a faraway look. "The first time I showed everyone at class, they even gave me a round of applause! Thinking back on it now, seeing things through like that and sweeping away what had been a pretty burdensome inferiority complex for me really got me motivated for the difficult task I faced in Osaka. That's why I'm so grateful to Eiko and to my yoga classmates."

Oba still found it hard to think of himself in Hori's position. "But Tetsuya, you're slim and you've always been good at sports. Isn't that the real reason you were able to accomplish the splits so easily?"

"You might think so," said Hori, "but according to Eiko just about anybody can learn to do the splits. Let's say you ran the one-hundred-meter dash today in a time of just under fifteen seconds. Frankly, the odds that you'd ever break the ten-second barrier are pretty slim no matter how hard you tried, right?"

"Well," said Oba, "I think that would be all but impossible."

"Sure," said Hori. "But even though the splits look incredibly hard, they actually don't require such a high level of athletic ability. Although there's individual variation, just about anyone can learn to do the splits as long as they stick to the program." Seeing that the others still had their doubts, he pressed on. "You know, overcoming your own complexes and having a more positive attitude aren't the only things to be gained by being able to do the splits. There are lots of other benefits, too."

As if he were giving a presentation about a new product, Hori began using a white board to list the positive effects of doing the splits:

1. Dieting

2. Better anti-aging and balance

3. Injury prevention

72

4. Toned legs less prone to swelling

5. Flatter belly

Note: Those with a misaligned pelvis or who have lower back, knee, or hip-joint pain should consult with a physician first.

Oba and Umemoto were amazed to see such a long list of appealing "side benefits" to doing the splits.

"Tetsuya," said Oba. "You did lose weight while you were in Osaka, didn't you? Meanwhile, my belly's starting to show. . . ."

"I lost ten pounds in the last two years," said Hori. "Everybody at the company seems to think I was just working myself to the bone turning around the Osaka branch, but it was actually thanks to doing the splits."

"You really do seem leaner than before," said Oba. "I could tell you somehow carried yourself with greater ease, but I never would have guessed your secret was doing the splits."

"Wow," said Umemoto. "There are so many benefits to doing the splits!"

As if he had been waiting for Umemoto's words, Hori turned again to face the others and said, "I know you both have a number of things that are bothering you. What do you think? It must have been some kind of fate that you happened to walk in on me like that. Do you want to try the four-week program and learn to do the splits?" Hori's tone was joking but his expression was completely serious.

"I don't know, Tetsuya," said Oba. "I'm not sure I could stick with it. Something tells me I wouldn't make it."

"Me, too," said Umemoto. "I've tried taking different kinds of lessons and going to sports clubs but I've never been able to see things through to the end."

"Look," Hori replied. "It isn't a matter of whether you're able to do it." He stood up. "The only thing that matters is whether you try. It isn't important whether you're good at it, or what you ultimately accomplish. The key is your attitude. At least that's what I believe."

Hori spoke with such conviction, and so convincingly, that Oba and Umemoto were both fired up.

"Okay, Tetsuya," said Oba. "Count me in."

"I'll do it, too!" added Umemoto.

"All right, then," said Hori. "I was pretty sure you'd say that. Listen, it's just the splits, but this isn't just going to loosen up your body. It will also change the way you feel. I guarantee it."

Oba and Umemoto found themselves once again drawn in by Hori's charisma. *Ah, so this is how he gets the most out of his subordinates, making them aware of a short-term objective and then setting them loose.* Oba felt as if he now understood why Hori had been so successful as a manager.

THE COMPLETE "SPLITS IN FOUR WEEKS" PROGRAM

"Okay," said Hori. "Let's start with an overview of the Splits in Four Weeks program that I learned from Eiko." He erased the white board and began to write down a description of the program.

The Splits in Four Weeks Program

• Basic Stretch 1: Towel Stretch

• Basic Stretch 2: Sumo Stretch

• Weekly Stretch x 4 Types

Week 1: Inner Thigh Stretch

Week 2: Wall Stretch

Week 3: Chair Stretch

Week 4: Door Stretch

• Achieve the Splits!

"First," said Hori, "being able to do the splits—that is, being able to spread your legs fully and place both elbows on the floor—boils down to loosening up the backs of your legs, your ankles, and your knees."

"You know, when we did that stretch a minute ago," said Oba, "I could really feel it working on the backs of my legs."

"Of course you could," said Hori. "Like I said, it all boils down to stretching out the backs of your legs. I'm going to explain the four-week program now, and I know you'll be able to see how logical and time-efficient the steps are. It's always better to see results sooner than later, right?"

Displaying her usual studious approach, Umemoto quickly took out a memo pad and began taking notes. "In other words," she said, "the program is made up of four week-long stages. Basic stretches one and two are common to each stage, supplemented by a different weekly stretch each time, right?"

"Exactly," said Hori. "You do three types of daily stretches each week. I'll go through all the details. We'll start with the two basic stretches, okay? Ai, do you want to try, too, this time?"

"Sure," Umemoto said. "Let me have a go."

"Okay! Makoto take this towel. We're going to start with the towel stretch, and afterward, I'll show you the sumo stretch."

A road of a thousand miles begins with one step.

−JAPANESE PROVERB

1 Towel Stretch

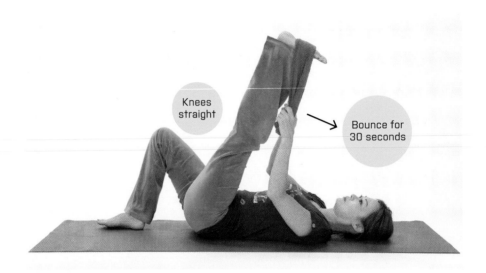

Knees
straight

Bounce for
30 seconds

Loop a hand towel over the underside of one foot, extend your leg (keeping your knee straight) and pull the towel toward your head with both hands, bouncing for 30 seconds. Do the same with the other leg.

Don't Do This

This is OK

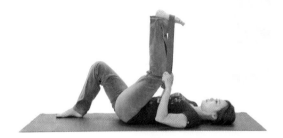

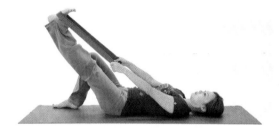

If you bend your knee, you won't get much of a stretch. If this stretch is difficult, use something longer like a bath towel, rope, or belt.

If this stretch is difficult, it's okay not to draw your leg closer. Just be sure to keep your knee straight.

2 Sumo Stretch

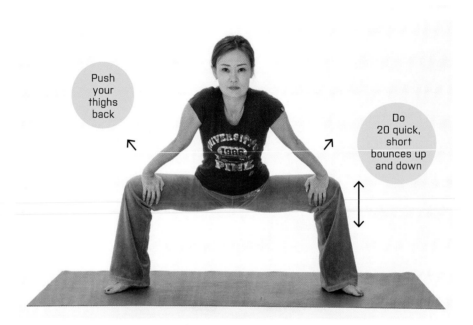

Push your thighs back

Do 20 quick, short bounces up and down

1 Point your knees outward, spread your legs about twice the width of your shoulders, lower your backside, and place your hands on your inner thighs near your knees. Your thighs should be parallel to the floor.

2 Bounce up and down in quick, short movements about 20 times.

3 Next, stretch the groin and back by twisting each shoulder toward the middle in turn while pushing harder with your hands.

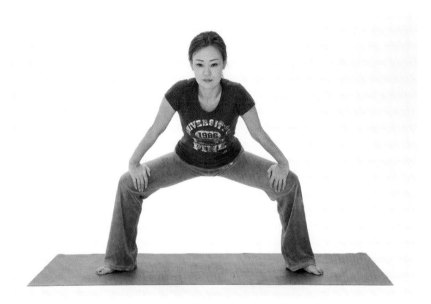

If this stretch is difficult, it's okay not
to lower your hips all the way.

"You'll repeat these two basic stretches every day until you're able to do the splits," Hori explained. "They act as benchmarks, too. As you get nearer to being able to do the splits, you'll see how you're able to draw your leg closer to your head during the towel stretch and lower your backside farther during the sumo stretch."

Oba was already breathing a little hard, but Umemoto seemed to be enjoying herself. "I see," she said. "Next we add the weekly stretches, right?"

"That's right. Here's the one for the first week."

Learning is like rowing upstream; not to advance is to drop back.

—JAPANESE PROVERB

Inner Thigh Stretch

In addition to the two basic stretches, you'll do one stretch that changes each week. For the first week, this is an inner thigh stretch. After you've finished each day's routine, be sure to try doing the splits.

BASIC STRETCHES TO DO EVERY DAY

1 Towel Stretch

2 Sumo Stretch

3 Inner Thigh Stretch

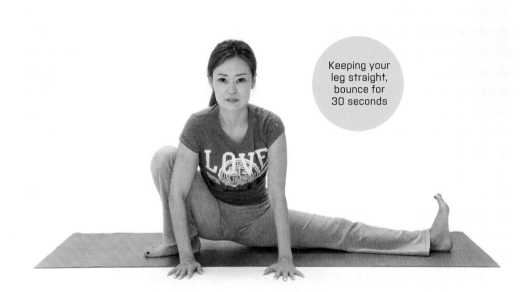

Keeping your leg straight, bounce for 30 seconds

With one knee bent, stretch out the other leg to the side, bouncing for 30 seconds. Do the same with the other leg.

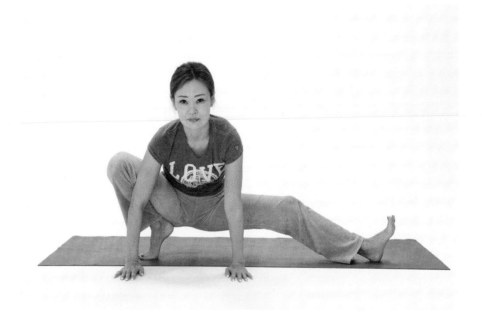

This stretch won't be effective if
both of your knees are bent.

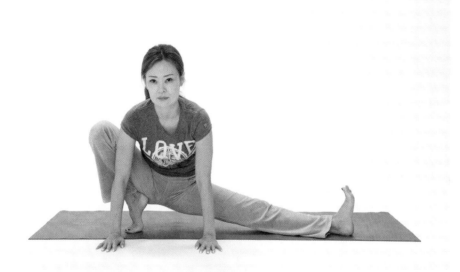

This is
is
OK

If you're inflexible, it's okay if the heel
of the bent leg leaves the floor.

When
you're
done with
week one,
try doing
the splits
to check
your
progress!

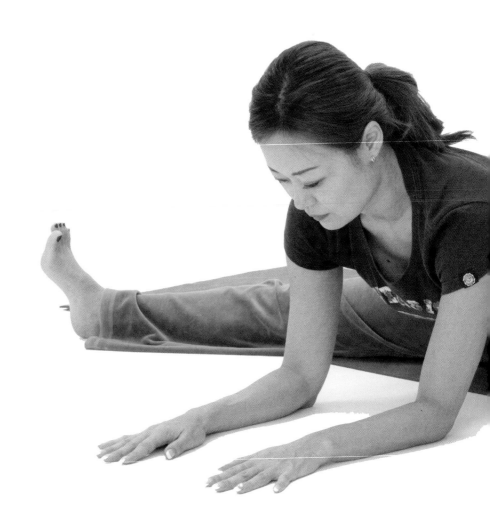

Sit with your legs spread out as far as they will go without bending your knees and lean your upper body forward. Your ultimate goal is for both elbows to touch the floor. Having someone photograph you each day from the same position is an easy way to track your progress. (You can also try taking pictures of yourself in a mirror.)

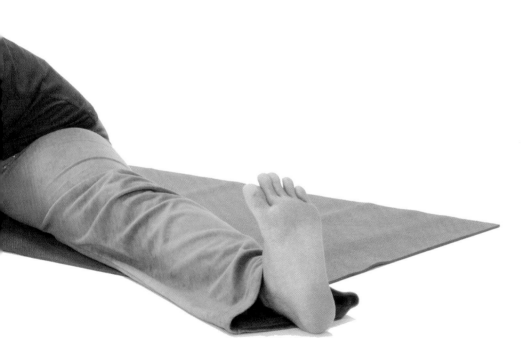

"You know, Tetsuya," said Oba. "This isn't particularly difficult, but it is kind of intense."

"I agree," said Umemoto. "But the fact that it's intense means it's working, right?"

"You're absolutely right, Ai," said Hori. "You're both starting out not very limber, so the first week is going to feel particularly intense. Okay, then. Let's review the main points."

Key Points and Cautions

- **Clothing** Wear loose clothing that makes it easy to move. Pants with elastic at the waist are best.

- **Location** Somewhat softer flooring is best. Putting down a blanket or yoga mat is optimal. Don't use beds because they are too soft.

- **Timing** After a bath or shower is best because the body is warm and more flexible.

- **Breathing** Exhale with a "haa" rather than a "hoo," as if expelling excess heat trapped inside the body.

Cautions: Whenever you stretch, be careful not to push yourself too hard. Injuring yourself is counterproductive. Instead of pushing yourself to your limit, aim for about 70 percent when you stretch. There is a tendency to push too hard when you're just starting out because you still can't do very much, but be careful because it is also easy to go too far once you begin to limber up and start to really enjoy the stretching.

"Got it?" Hori asked. "And one last thing. Your goal at the end of four weeks is to be able to sit on the floor with your legs spread and lean your upper body forward so that both elbows touch the floor." He demonstrated his own split one more time, spreading his legs fully, lowering his upper body effortlessly, and placing both elbows on the floor.

"Amazing, Tetsuya," said Oba. "So that's what we need to aim for, then?"

"Right. I can bring my whole upper body all the way down to the floor like a pancake, and this is generally enough for people to recognize you've done the splits."

"It sure is," said Umemoto. "You move so smoothly, just like a gymnast."

"Thanks," said Hori. "I think that's enough for today. I'll go over the stretches for week two and beyond another time. Any questions?"

"Tetsuya," said Oba, "as you can see, I've gained a little weight. Is that going to be a problem for doing the splits?

"Not at all," said Hori. "Eiko says to think about sumo wrestlers. They all do *matawari* training, which is a lot like straddle splits, and most of them weigh a whole lot more than 200 pounds. In other words, whether you can do the splits, and whether you're flexible or not, has nothing to do with how much you weigh or how fat or skinny your legs are."

Oba nodded.

"Okay," said Hori, smiling broadly. "Let's reconvene here in a week and see what kind of progress you've made. Good luck to you both. That's all for today!"

"Okay!" answered Oba and Umemoto together, their expressions conveying their motivation.

A CHALLENGING START

"I can't believe it!" Trying to lift his leg toward the ceiling, Oba ended up raising his voice instead of his leg. Not only did it hurt, he was also shocked at how inflexible his body had become.

On Tuesday he had arrived home early after work, eaten a quick dinner, had a bath, then laid out a blanket on the floor to do his towel stretch.

Oba thought back to the first time he met Hori, when he was 21 and Hori came back to campus as a recruiter. They had met at a coffee shop near the office, one that was no longer in business, and for some reason ordered melon floats. Hori had cheerfully told him all about the work he was doing at the time. Oba didn't think twice about making the company his first choice.

Ever since then, Hori had always been someone who walked a few steps ahead, a mentor he could look up to. This had always seemed perfectly natural, something not even worth questioning. Until now, he had never stopped to think about why Hori was so great, had never dug deeper to think about what enabled him to always shine.

Maybe it would have been different had he and Hori entered the company at the same time, but the fact that Hori was older—and it was expected that he would be more accomplished—had prevented him from thinking further about the reasons Hori was so amazing.

Now he was going to experience for himself what made his mentor great. This was Oba's other reason for wanting to master the splits.

"Ugh, Ow!"

This wasn't going to easy, though. Even after being taught how to do the stretches, once he started doing them himself he was no longer sure he was doing them right. His body had not yet internalized what he had heard.

He was using a long bath towel for the towel stretch. He had tried using a hand towel at first, but that was too big a leap to make right from the outset. After switching to a bath towel, he struggled to figure out how far to stretch and ended up going too far.

STRETCHES LIKE THE SPLITS CAN PREVENT INJURIES

By doing the splits, you're increasing your muscle strength, flexibility, and range of motion. Studies even show that targeted lower body stretching significantly increases range of motion in other areas of the body like the shoulders and upper body.[9]

People who don't exercise much (or not at all) are more prone to injuries. Their stiff bodies aren't conditioned for or comfortable with unfamiliar movements that can happen when the body moves in unexpected or accidental ways like during a stumble or fall. By doing the splits, you're making your body familiar with a whole range of uncommon movements, which helps you resist injury, and can even speed up recovery from injuries.[10] (See page 103 for more info on the negative effects of a sedentary lifestyle.)

Even if you do exercise frequently, you can benefit from practicing the splits. Stretching helps prevent exercise-related injury, improves your physical performance,[11] and reduces post exercise muscle soreness.[12]

Next he tried the sumo stretch, but couldn't get his backside down at all. He would never have imagined that in this way he would gain a newfound respect for the sumo wrestlers he saw on television.

"Hey, Dad. What are you doing? Sumo?" On his way to bed, Tsubasa peeked in curiously, not having missed the sudden change in his father. "I want to play, too!" Following Oba's example, he started doing the sumo stretch. He was able to lower his backside a lot farther than Oba. Kids' bodies really are limber. "Good night, Dad," he said. "Don't hurt yourself this time, okay?"

His son's words stung. *One of these days I'll show you some awesome dribbling again!* Still, his present condition was pretty pathetic. Was this really going to help him do the splits?

An hour later, having returned home after staying a bit late at work to revise her presentation for Hori, Umemoto ate dinner and had a bath, then pulled her yoga mat from the back of her closet where it had been tucked away for a while.

She had never imagined that the expensive yoga mat would actually prove useful one day. Wanting to look the part, she had splurged on it when she started the yoga classes that she ended up abandoning after just a few sessions.

For the towel stretch she wasn't even able to get her legs to forty-five degrees. For the sumo stretch, she not only couldn't get her backside down at all, her everyday lack of exercise left her legs shaking terribly. She knew in her mind that it was important to stretch, but it was hard to take a positive attitude when she felt so miserable and scared.

What was more, at this point she didn't have any sense that she was actually getting any closer to the goal. She had known she was inflexible, but never realized how bad it really was. Umemoto felt terrible. It was hard to remember why she had wanted to try to do the splits in the first place.

It was hard enough for her living alone, but she imagined it would be even worse for Oba. What if his family laughed at him when he suddenly started stretching?

The next day, Umemoto quickly found Oba and asked him candidly how things had gone. "Makoto," she said. "How did you do?"

"In a word, terrible," he said. "My son started doing impressions and my wife laughed at me."

"I was afraid that might happen. How are we ever going to get to the point where it feels like we're getting closer to doing the splits? At this rate, it just feels like some kind of austere religious ritual."

Hori noticed the two of them chatting and approached with a smile. "Hey, you two. No more of this talking about personal stuff on company time."

"Tetsuya," said Oba, "how did you know what we were talking about?"

"Well," Hori replied, "it's written all over your faces: 'Enough, already.'"

"Uh-oh. He's seen right through us, hasn't he, Makoto?" The confidence Umemoto had exhibited in the conference room on Monday was gone.

"I'm pretty sure I mentioned this before," said Hori, "but the toughest part is when you're just getting started. Why don't you both just focus on getting through this phase, on sticking to it every day?"

"I suppose you're right," said Umemoto. "But it's hard not having any sense that we're getting closer to the goal."

"I see," said Hori. "You know, there are a number of ways you can track your progress. For example, you could use the standing forward bend that we did at the beginning to monitor how much more flexible your body is getting, or do the same thing with the seated forward bend, where you lean your upper body forward and try to grab your ankles. It may seem crude, but you could even tape a ruler to the wall, measure your results every day, and put the numbers in a graph to visualize your progress. You're good at that sort of thing, aren't you, Ai?"

"Yes, I am," she said.

"It wouldn't be a bad idea to use your smartphone to record yourself, either," continued Hori. "If you always do your stretches in the same place, and set up your phone in the same location, you'll be able to see your progress as you gain flexibility from one day to the next. Makoto, you must have a video camera lying around for recording your son playing soccer, right?"

"Yes, I do."

"It's important to use tools like that so you can get a sense of your progress and stay motivated. Once you become a businessperson, there aren't very many chances to physically experience how difficult it is to keep up with something. Why not feel grateful for the opportunity?"

That was just like his mentor. Oba was reminded again what a great leader Hori was.

"Hey, that reminds me," said Hori, "I wanted to let you know that Eiko's going to be in Tokyo next Monday to give a talk. I thought I would take her out for a meal to thank her for everything and wondered if you two might like to come along and meet her."

"Wow," said Umemoto. "That would be great!"

"Really?" said Oba. "You think we'll get some hints right from the source?"

"Maybe," said Hori. "I'll have her stop by the office, then. Don't forget to bring a change of clothes, okay?"

MEETING THE QUEEN OF SPLITS

(Explanation of Week 2)

The following Monday they all met in the conference room as promised to measure Oba and Umemoto's results after completing their first week. Both were clearly able to reach farther than they had the week before.

"Okay," said Hori. "You've made it through the hardest part: the first week! You've made real progress toward doing the splits. Keep up the good work."

Oba and Umemoto both beamed, but Oba enjoyed Hori's words for another reason, too. His mentor had always had a way of doling out praise, and he knew Hori was probably laying it on a little thick on purpose. He did it with such warmth, though, that it didn't feel obvious.

Oba was glad to have Hori back in Tokyo, and to be trying—however unexpectedly—to overcome his own lack of flexibility. It was good to have his trusted mentor nearby again.

Hori's mobile phone rang. Eiko had arrived at the receptionist's desk. Oba and Umemoto, who had already changed their clothes, stayed in the conference room while Hori went off on his own to show her in.

"Makoto," said Umemoto. "Director Hori is really good at giving praise, isn't he? I mean, just talking with him makes me want to work even harder."

"I know," Oba replied. "He's always been like that."

Hori and Eiko entered the room. To Oba and Umemoto, Eiko looked even slimmer than she did in her popular video. "How nice to meet you," she said. "Tetsuya's two favorite students."

"Hi, I'm Makoto. Thanks so much for helping us out tonight."

"And I'm Ai. Eiko, you're so slender!"

"Well, thank you," said Eiko. "If I were overweight, nobody would believe me when I said doing the splits helped with dieting. I actually do love to eat, though."

Hori explained what Oba and Umemoto had done so far and asked her to provide some advice. Eiko started off by explaining the fundamentals of the stretches.

"You know," she began. "Being inflexible and unable to do the splits is just a matter of tension in the hip joints and the surrounding muscles. The stretches you've been doing in your first week are designed to loosen that area up. Pretty intense, aren't they?"

"Yes," said Oba. "To tell you the truth, I thought it was going to kill me."

"I couldn't get used to it," added Umemoto, "and nearly gave up."

"I know what you mean," said Eiko. "Now I teach as if I were an expert, but I used to be really stiff. I became an instructor despite not being very limber myself."

"Hard to believe, isn't it?" said Hori. "But it's true. Listen, since Eiko's here, why don't we have her show you what a really beautiful split looks like?"

Urged on by Hori, Eiko finished changing her clothes and demonstrated the splits of a pro.

"Wow," said Oba. "Out of this world."

"Beautiful," said Umemoto. "You're so graceful, almost birdlike."

After the two of them had cheered and sighed, Eiko stood up and began to talk.

"Being able to do the splits may look beautiful and seem impressive, but more than that it also has lots of other benefits. Surely, Tetsuya must have told you about them?"

"Yes," said Hori. "I went through the basics, but please, why don't you describe them in more detail yourself?"

"The first thing," said Eiko, "is dieting. Keeping up with the stretches that you do to accomplish the splits loosens up your body, which raises your basal metabolic rate and improves circulation. You can even expect an anti-aging effect. Just look at Tetsuya."

"Ah, so the splits are your secret to looking so ageless," said Oba, looking convinced.

"Ai," asked Eiko, "do you ever suffer from sensitivity to the cold?"

"I do. In the winter, of course, but the air conditioning here at the office runs pretty strong during the summer, too. Right, Makoto?"

"Better circulation will help with your sensitivity to cold," said Eiko, "so maybe this summer you won't have to argue with Makoto about where to set the temperature."

"And since I'll be losing weight at the same time," said Oba with a wry grin, "I'm sure I'll be fine with a higher temperature."

"Next," continued Eiko, "is preventing injury. The more flexible someone is, the less likely they are to get injured while playing sports. Having stiff knees and hip joints can lead to muscle strains in your thighs."

"Hey, Makoto," said Umemoto, "That sounds like what happened to you."

"That's right," he said. "The other day I was playing soccer with my son and as soon as I started taking it seriously I ended up taking a tumble."

"As you get closer to being able to do the splits," said Eiko, "I'm sure you'll see things improve. But you know, Ai, as a woman you may benefit the most from doing the splits."

"Really?"

"Improved circulation reduces swelling of your legs and tightens them up, while shifting your hip joints back into place helps fix bowlegs and knock-knees. Being more limber also corrects any misalignment and ensures that your spine sits properly on your pelvis. That brings your upper and lower body into balance, which makes your body more stable and tightens your tummy."

"Wow," exclaimed Umemoto. "That all sounds wonderful!" Then, in a softer voice, she added, "You know, I've actually got bowlegs."

"In that case," said Eiko, "the sumo stretch will be especially helpful. That stretch was originally designed for injury prevention, but it's also the reason you never see bowlegged sumo wrestlers."

"You're right," interrupted Oba. "I've never seen a sumo wrestler with bowlegs."

"As your hip joints loosen up, it also lengthens your stride, which is good for people who run," said Eiko. "Oh, and it can keep you from slipping, too, Makoto."

"You got me," he said. "I'm just glad I didn't really hurt myself last week."

"You two are both learning a lot, aren't you?" said Hori, looking satisfied. "Eiko, could you tell these two why you're so sure that anyone can learn to do the splits?"

"Of course," she replied. "The simplest reason is that all of you probably used to be able to do the splits without even trying. That means you, Makoto, and you, too, Ai."

"Really?" said Umemoto. "I've never been good at sports and don't remember anything like that."

"Exactly," said Eiko. "It was back before you can remember. All human babies start out with hip joints that rotate three hundred sixty degrees. You know how flexible babies are, right?"

"You're right," said Oba. "My son Tsubasa was so floppy he used to sleep with his legs splayed out to the side like a frog."

"But at about the age of three," Eiko continued, "the joints that you don't move—both the joints themselves and the muscles around them—start to tighten up. With the hip joints being able to walk and run is enough—there's no need to rotate them completely—so their range of motion narrows. This tendency is particularly strong in people like you, who maintain the same posture during much of their time on the job. Sitting or driving or working at a computer all the time not only leads to soreness, but it also tightens up the joints. In other words, the instant your body stops moving, it starts to get stiff. And the same holds true for all your joints."

"But Eiko," said Umemoto, "some people are just naturally flexible, aren't they?"

"Yes. Everybody's joints stiffen up over time, but the pace varies from person to person and there are some people whose joints remain flexible even though they don't exercise at all. People like

AVOID THE DREADED "SITTING DISEASE" WITH THE SPLITS!

"Sitting disease" has recently been coined as a type of umbrella term by the scientific community to account for the various maladies caused by days of seated commutes, office jobs, and returning home only to laze on the couch. It's no secret that a sedentary lifestyle can make hips stiff. Not only is this uncomfortable, it can also potentially lead to injury and even disability. Stretching is an ideal way to strengthen these super important body parts. "Strong hips are a must for even the most basic activities in life, such as walking," says Robert Turner, PT, OCS, a board-certified orthopedic specialist and clinical supervisor at the Spine Therapy Center at the Weill-Cornell affiliated Hospital for Special Surgery, in an article for Women's Nutrition Connection. "Your hips transfer forces from your upper body into the ground and from your legs up into your trunk as you're moving," Turner explains. "Weak hips will interfere with the transfer, essentially disconnecting your upper body from your lower body." He goes on to say that this affects "your gait, posture, and endurance." But stretching is a viable solution and leads not only to greater flexibility and effortless and uninhibited movement but an overall better quality of life.[13]

that are able to do the splits after just stretching a little bit. But even people who are inflexible have nothing to worry about. We were all flexible as babies, and people who are inflexible just have to work a little harder to bring back their old, limber bodies."

Oba suddenly decided to ask a question that had been on his mind. "I've known Tetsuya for a long time, and I can clearly see there's a new lightness in the way he carries himself. You're his secret, aren't you, Eiko?"

"Well, Tetsuya really worked hard," said Eiko. "When your body limbers up, it's only natural that you carry yourself more beautifully. It gets easier to step over things, to crouch, to stand, to pick things up. There probably aren't many people who set out with that as a goal, but it is one of the happy by-products of being able to do the splits."

Glancing at the clock, Hori said, "Hey, I've made the reservation for eight o'clock. We can keep the conversation going at the restaurant, but could you show these two the wall stretch before we go?"

"Sure," said Eiko.

The bamboo that bends is stronger than the oak that resists.

–JAPANESE PROVERB

The weekly stretch for week two uses a wall to bring you closer to the splits. Since the wall supports the weight of your legs, you can increase the intensity without bending your knees and without pushing too far.

BASIC STRETCHES TO DO EVERY DAY

1 Towel Stretch

2 Sumo Stretch

3 Wall Stretch

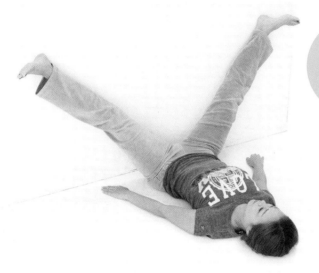

Stretch for
1 to 2 minutes
while
bouncing

1 Position your backside along the wall, extend your legs toward the ceiling, then open up your legs.

2 Place your legs against the wall, spread them as far as you can without bending your knees or pushing too far, and stretch for 1 to 2 minutes while bouncing.

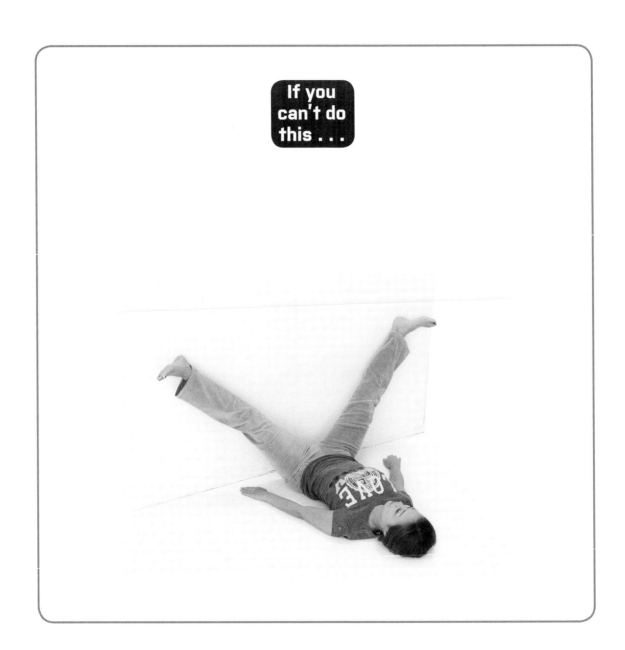

If you
can't do
this . . .

This
is
OK

Adjust the intensity of the stretch by varying how open your legs are and the distance between your backside and the wall. If this stretch is difficult, it's okay to only go as far as you can.

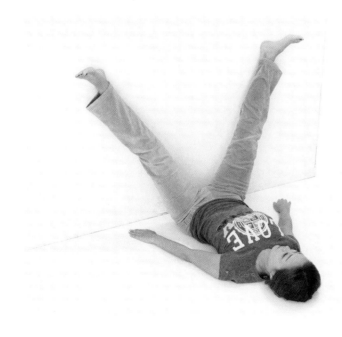

When you're done with week two, try doing the splits to check your progress!

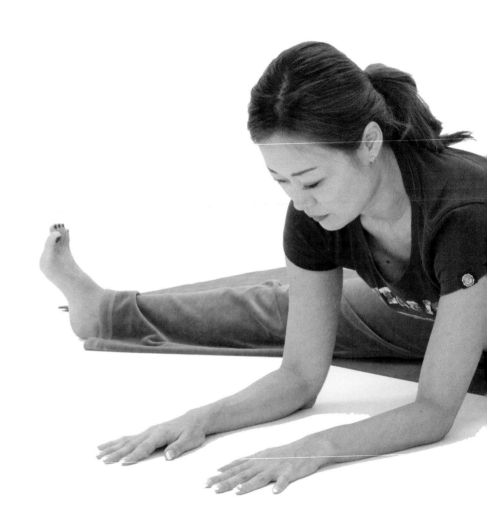

Sit with your legs spread out as far as they will go without bending your knees and lean your upper body forward. Your ultimate goal is for both elbows to touch the floor. Having someone photograph you each day from the same position is an easy way to track your progress. (You can also try taking pictures of yourself in a mirror.)

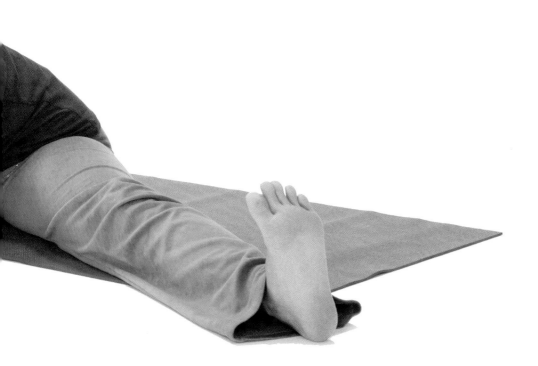

The four of them arrived at a restaurant near the office that Hori had often used before, one where Oba knew the chef, too. Over dinner and drinks, their conversation about the splits continued to flow, with Umemoto a particularly enthusiastic participant.

"Eiko," she said, "I can't help feeling nervous about going too far when I'm doing the stretches. What should I do?"

"It isn't good to push yourself too hard. I overstretched and hurt myself once when I was working on yoga, and I can tell you that overstretching is completely counterproductive. The point is to get healthier, right? So it's a good thing to feel a little bit apprehensive; that's a sign you've gone far enough and shouldn't overdo it."

"I see," said Umemoto. "But how can I tell how much is the right amount to stretch?"

"The first thing to do," Eiko replied, "is to make sure you warm up properly. In my four-week program, the towel stretch and sumo stretch actually serve as your warm-ups."

"Ah," said Umemoto. "That makes sense."

Oba leaned forward to listen more closely. As he understood more about the program, he could feel himself getting more motivated.

"The important thing," said Eiko, "is that if one hundred percent represents the maximum you can possibly stretch, you should always stop at what feels like about seventy percent. That's right about where it starts to hurt in a good way. Going any farther is too far. You should definitely avoid going so far that it makes you catch your breath."

"Eiko," said Umemoto, "speaking of breathing, Director Hori said we should exhale with a 'haa' sound rather than a 'hoo.' Why is that?"

"Because it helps expel heat. If you exhale with a 'hoo' or a 'shoo' sound, your breath is cool, but if you exhale with a 'haa,' it's warm, right? Try it."

Everyone exhaled with a "haa."

"Hey, you're right!"

"Come to think of it, when it's cold outside in the winter, nobody tries to warm their hands by blowing 'hoo.' It's always 'haa,' isn't it?"

"Right," said Eiko. "In the yoga world this is called the Breath of Fire. You can increase your flexibility effectively without hurting yourself by exhaling with a 'haa.'"

"Okay," said Umemoto. "Not 'hoo,' 'haa.' Not 'hoo,' 'haa.'" She repeated the phrase so many times, earnestly checking to see that she had it right, that the others were amused.

Hori urged Eiko to continue. "You often suggest bouncing the body when stretching. That's another basic technique, isn't it?"

"Yes, that's right," replied Eiko. "It's better to bounce a little bit. This stimulates the entire muscle, loosening while stretching in a way that feels good. Bouncing also ensures you don't stretch too far, so it even helps prevent injury. In my four-week program, the two basic stretches—the towel stretch and the sumo stretch, as well as the inner thigh stretch in week one and the door stretch in week four— are all more effective if done with a little bounce."

The time passed quickly as the group enjoyed the delicious food, but the conversation showed no sign of letting up. Oba decided to ask something that had been bothering him. "Eiko," he said, "the fact is, sometimes I worry whether I'll really ever be able to do the splits. I know this is kind of vague, but do you have any advice?"

"That's all right," said Eiko. "I've been there myself, so I know what you mean. Let's see. I've taught a lot of people, and I suppose the biggest reason some people give up is that it starts to feel like a chore. The issue really doesn't have anything to do with technical aspects of stretching or the splits. It's more a matter of attitude."

"I see," said Oba. "Tetsuya did say it was a matter of whether or not you try."

"After all," said Eiko, "one of my students learned to do a complete pancake split at the age of seventy-two."

"Really?" Oba and Umemoto both blurted out simultaneously.

"Really," said Eiko. "Yes, there's some individual variation, but most people who apply themselves manage to do the splits in a month, and anyone can do it if they spend a little more time. You don't have to be a former gymnast or to have trained in ballet. The splits rewards those who don't give up. I guarantee it!"

Oba and Umemoto felt encouraged by her reassuring words.

"You know," said Eiko. "I think whether you can do the splits is actually something bigger than just the splits. It's a matter of whether you can succeed at something you set your mind to, whether you can set the course of your life on your own."

Hori nodded deeply.

"Even if it isn't directly related," Eiko continued, "I think the splits are an effective way to develop a positive mind-set—the feeling that you can do anything. I don't have any evidence for this, of course, but I'm pretty sure Tetsuya knows what I mean."

"I agree," said Hori. "That's why I wanted these two to experience it, too. Eiko, I hope you'll continue to share your advice with them."

Eiko gave the others a number of hints for sticking with the program and not giving up:

- That even if they were really busy, they should still be sure to stretch for at least a minute.

- That if they were really short of time, they should prioritize the sumo stretch.

- That even if they didn't see progress on any given day, they should try at least to maintain the results of the day before to avoid slipping backward.

- That although it was ideal to set clear goals and reach them one by one, in the real world the most important thing was to find a way to stay motivated, even when things were difficult.

- That it was important to maintain a steady pace and not rush on ahead when they were feeling good.

- That the approach was a lot like the one used for successful diets.

Eiko also told them that the idea that drinking alcohol would loosen up their bodies was nothing but an urban legend and had no basis in fact. Hori and Oba recalled how they had heard that circus performers all remained limber by drinking vinegar, another urban legend that seemed to have fallen out of favor before Umemoto's time.

Before the evening ended, Eiko told them something else that was interesting. "When I do the splits, I find that I sometimes get so wound up that it feels good even though it hurts, or I get so relaxed that it feels like I might fall asleep. It's like a kind of high, and feels really good."

"Really?" Both Oba and Umemoto looked as if they found this hard to believe, which was unsurprising given that for now they both felt the program was pretty harsh.

"I call it the 'splits high,'" said Eiko. "You know, just like a runner's high or a climber's high. I'm sure the same thing applies to the splits. That's why whenever I get worried or have something to think about, I do the splits."

"I know what you mean," said Hori, who seemed to recognize the feeling. "It clears your head and opens the way for good ideas. That's why I want the two of you to feel what it's like. Doing the stretches and the splits isn't all agony, you know. Just three more weeks—stick with it!"

STICKING WITH IT IS HARD

(Week 2 in Practice)

"Not good, Umemoto. This would have been really humiliating if we hadn't caught it in time. I don't understand, though. It isn't like you to make careless mistakes like this." Scolded by her immediate superior, Umemoto felt terribly small. She had always taken pride in error-free work and wasn't accustomed to being called out for making mistakes.

Umemoto and Oba were in the same department but in different sections. The section manager to whom Umemoto reported had asked her to analyze a new client and prepare documentation for a proposal, but it was a field she had not previously researched and had taken her longer than expected. Some issues then came up with an existing client, she ran out of time, and she missed some things during final revisions.

And that wasn't all. She had accidentally mistyped one of the numbers in the tabulated data, leading to misplaced conclusions and a proposal that was completely off the mark. Her manager had caught the mistake before it went out, which was a good thing for the company.

Umemoto knew what the problem was. No matter how busy she had been at work, she had been sure to make time to do her splits stretches. Given how much she aspired to be like Hori, and how serious Oba—who always looked out for her—was taking things, there was no way she could throw in the towel.

Following Eiko's teaching and advice, she had made sure to always at least do the sumo stretch, no matter how tired and groggy she was. Still, with so many new things all piling up at once, she had made the sort of mistake for which she could not forgive herself. Umemoto lost confidence completely.

For Oba, the organizational reshuffle and new responsibilities resulted in a succession of unavoidable after-five commitments with colleagues and clients, and he ended up going out drinking a lot. Although he had never been a big drinker, his position at work required him to keep up with the others. Getting up to speed on his new role slowed his progress in clearing away ordinary desk work and took time from briefing others on his old duties, so that, even on the days when he expected to get home early, he found it a challenge to get away from the office.

On Friday, he barely made the last train as it was leaving the station, and then the service was further delayed by an accident on the line. He got home so late that he ended up skipping his stretches that night, falling asleep before he knew it.

Actually, just before drifting off to sleep at the limits of consciousness, he had been aware for a moment that he was going to miss his stretches.

If only he could be more like Hori.

If only he could carry himself so smoothly both at work and in his private life.

His wife and Tsubasa would sure be surprised if he were able to do the splits.

He might even be able to get back on the soccer team, and play with Tsubasa all he wanted.

Oba didn't think that asking for all these things would be asking too much. He was sure Hori would be able to accomplish them all without a hitch.

It was this sense of impatience that pushed Oba to stretch more than necessary. The day before, while spreading his legs to do the wall stretch, he had been so pleased to see how much easier it was to do than it had been on Monday that he had ended up stretching himself beyond his limit.

He thought he was maintaining his limit, legs up against the wall, when carelessness, declining muscle strength, and gravity suddenly combined to pull his legs open to 110 percent.

"Ow!" He cried out so shrilly that his sleeping wife woke up in surprise.

So that Oba and Umemoto could stay in touch with Eiko in Osaka, Hori had set up an online group for the four of them. The next day, Saturday, Eiko sent Umemoto the following advice:

Hello, Ai. It sounds like you've had a rough week at work. The reason to keep stretching every day isn't to push yourself unreasonably. You won't be able to stick with the splits if you push so hard that it gets in the way of your work and your life. It's just like dieting: if you cut down on what you eat and drink so much that you're too weak to go to work, you lose everything. Sticking with the stretching every day is a way of developing the self-control you need to keep it up every day.

She also sent the following message to Oba:

Makoto, you've had a hard week at the office, haven't you? How are you feeling? It's best to stretch after a bath and before you go to bed, but when things come up or you've been out drinking and that isn't possible, consider going to sleep and then stretching when you get up. There's no reason to push yourself so hard that you hurt yourself.

Let me give you some advice, just in case you do get hurt. Unless you are really injured, it's counterproductive to stop stretching just because of a little pain. Keep at it every day, stretching to about 60 percent. The improved circulation should help you heal faster, while not stretching because it hurts will actually slow down your recovery. Whatever happens, just don't overdo it.

Hori was impressed with Eiko's compassionate advice, and knew that all he could do now was add his encouragement as well:

You two are doing great! I've been so busy lately I'm sorry I haven't had time to be much help either with work or with the splits. I've made sure to leave Monday evening open, though, so you can fill me in then.

Eiko then sent a message of further support:

This reminds me of when Tetsuya was working hard on the splits two years ago. He always applied himself, both at home and at yoga class, though I knew he had other important things on his mind. There were times when he was so busy with work that he couldn't come to the studio, but he never made excuses and always came back.

He always kept a positive attitude, seeming to focus only on what he needed to do in any given situation to get better results. The other students and I became real fans and always tried to be supportive.

This was a side of Hori in Osaka that Oba and Umemoto had never seen. Having gradually gotten more comfortable, Umemoto wrote:

Eiko, I didn't tell Director Hori I was going to ask this, but was he popular at your studio? Most of your students are women, right?

Eiko replied:

Well, everyone had a lot of respect for him. Idolized him, almost. When he returned to Tokyo we all went to Shin Osaka station to see him off with a cheer.

Oba started to feel energized enough to break into the conversation.

No kidding? Wow, Tetsuya, maybe they all mistook you for some celebrity!

Grateful for everything Eiko had done, Hori confidently replied:

Amazing, huh? It really felt like being a star. And you two will be stars soon, too!

STRETCHING TONES YOUR LEGS— AND CUTS DOWN ON SWELLING

When you use your body weight for resistance, you're building up lean muscle that boosts your metabolism. Stretching develops strength, muscular endurance, and suppleness—all qualities which contribute to conditioning.[14]

Additionally, stretching has been proven to significantly aid healthy circulation.[15] Tight, inflexible muscles can hinder bloodflow, causing swelling and making muscles even more stiff. With regular stretching, you are improving your bloodflow and circulation and reducing painful swelling.[16]

HOW ARE YOU EVER GOING TO ACHIEVE ANYTHING IF YOU CAN'T EVEN DO THE SPLITS?

(Explanation of Week 3)

Monday evening rolled around again. It was time for Oba and Umemoto to try the standing forward bend and the splits after completing the wall stretches of week two. Concerned about their progress, Eiko checked in through their online group via video.

"How about it, Makoto?" asked Hori. "Does it still hurt? It's okay to take it slow."

Oba had followed Eiko's advice and taken it easy with his stretching on Saturday and Sunday. The pain was almost gone.

From Hori's perspective, both Oba and Umemoto seemed to have made a lot of progress toward being able to do the splits. He watched the videos that each had taken of themselves, which showed they had come a long way in the past two weeks. Oba's video showed his son Tsubasa earnestly watching over him, no longer making fun of his father.

"All right," said Hori. "I know this has been hard for you two, both physically and what with trying to balance it with work, but you've held up well and made real progress, haven't you?" he said encouragingly. "I'm really happy to see such visible results."

Not to be outdone, Eiko piped up from Osaka. "Terrific! Week three will be easier and more fun than week two, and week four more than week three. Once you've made it this far, the splits are nearly within reach. Good luck!"

"Okay," said Hori. "Let me explain the chair stretch for week three. Eiko, be sure to jump in if I miss anything, okay?"

3

Chair Stretch

For week three, you'll do a chair stretch, which applies pressure to your hip joints. The key is that the back of the chair enables you to freely adjust the intensity.

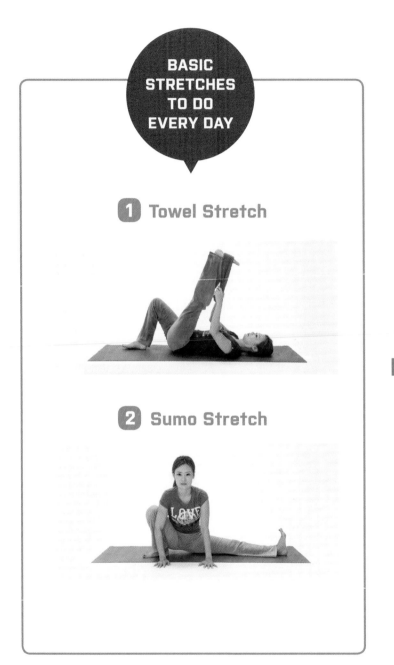

BASIC STRETCHES TO DO EVERY DAY

1 Towel Stretch

2 Sumo Stretch

+

❸ Chair Stretch

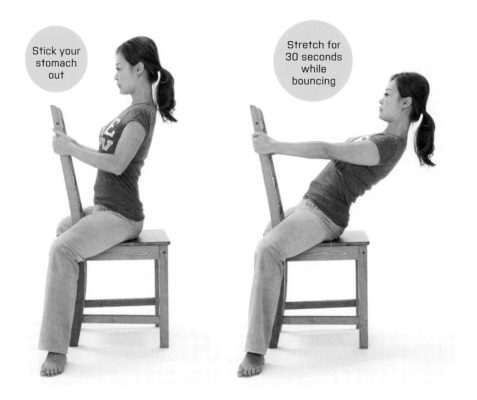

Stick your stomach out

Stretch for 30 seconds while bouncing

1 Straddle the chair facing the seat back with your feet in line with the back of the chair. Grabbing the seat back with both hands, stick your stomach out.

2 Lean your upper body back while pulling on the seat back, open up your knees, and stretch your hips for 30 seconds while bouncing.

When you're done with week three, try doing the splits to check your progress!

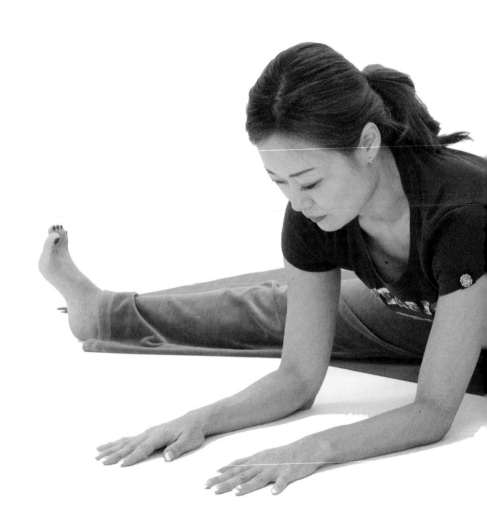

Sit with your legs spread out as far as they will go without bending your knees and lean your upper body forward. Your ultimate goal is for both elbows to touch the floor. Having someone photograph you each day from the same position is an easy way to track your progress. (You can also try taking pictures of yourself in a mirror.)

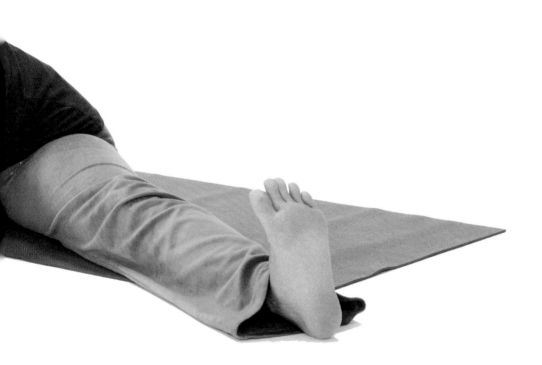

"Tetsuya, that was amazing!" Eiko was pleased with the way Hori had presented the stretch. "You could have a second career as an instructor!"

"Oh, I don't know," said Hori. "I may have overdone it a bit, knowing you were watching. But this does remind me a lot of two years ago. You really helped me so much then, and it's thanks to you that my posting in Osaka turned out to be so productive. Since our company benefited so much, it really ought to find a way to reward you!"

Eiko modestly deflected Hori's praise, said good-bye, and ended her call.

"Tetsuya," said Oba, his eyes shining. "I think I'm finally beginning to see how doing the splits meant something more to you than just overcoming a teenage inferiority complex."

"Me, too," said Umemoto, her analytical abilities having returned. "Maybe this is overstating the point, but it seems like the success you've had at the company, which everyone had been talking about, might be related to your success in doing the splits."

Hori turned to them both and slowly began to speak. "At a time when I felt like I could get crushed, I learned the importance of accepting new things, the powerful sensation of being able to do something I couldn't do before, and the motivation to take on new challenges. For me, it just happened to be the splits that triggered this."

Oba and Umemoto were a bit surprised to see how serious Hori's expression was.

"It isn't as if being able to do the splits means all that much," Hori continued. "But just as the two of you have experienced, it's surprising to see someone who can do the splits, isn't it? That sparkle you feel, that sense of respect—at least the way I see it—is something you reserve for the kind of people who keep on trying to accomplish something that most people can't."

"Tetsuya," asked Oba, "what kept you from quitting?"

"I wanted to step away from this idea that the company had sent me off on a lonely mission, or that I'd arrived in Osaka carrying everyone else's expectations and anxieties, and just focus on what I was going to do, on how I was going to proceed.

"I wanted people at the branch office to understand that it wasn't a matter of what other people thought, or the outside environment, or the direction of the economy. . . . Well, yes, these things are not completely unrelated, but they aren't the things you should be thinking about first. That's why I kept working on the splits, and was able to keep going without giving up."

Oba and Umemoto held their breath.

"So if the two of you aren't interested in the splits, it doesn't matter if you quit," Hori continued. "Needless to say, even if you do, it isn't going to lower your performance evaluation or reduce your bonus. If you hadn't peeked into the conference room two weeks ago, we probably wouldn't even be here today."

He was right, of course.

"But," Hori continued, "at the same time, I can see so clearly that it hurts that you've both hit a wall as you try to figure out where to go in your work and your lives. This isn't a bad thing at all. It's actually just like doing the splits. It's just the splits, but it's more than the splits. It's just a job, but it's more than a job. It's just living, but it's more than living." Then Hori took a deep breath and said, "How are you ever going to achieve anything if you can't even do the splits?"

THE WAY OF THE SPLITS

(Week 3 in Practice)

Oba and Umemoto started off again with a new stretch for the week. They no longer felt lost. Just as Eiko had said, they could feel it becoming easier, and more fun, to do the splits.

Oba's wife helped by pulling his arms during the pair stretch. Tsubasa tried to follow her example and help, too, but unfortunately he didn't have the necessary strength yet. The fact that he had tried to help at all, though, made Oba feel even more motivated to carry on.

Umemoto tried to find free moments to stretch as much as she could during work. Staring at the computer all day inevitably caused her body to tighten up and kept good ideas from coming to mind. At times like that she would find a chair at an open desk or in a conference room to stretch even if just for a minute. This loosened up her body and, surprisingly, provided a refreshing change of pace that made her work go more smoothly.

On Friday evening, after the two of them had sent a progress update to their online group as always, Eiko sent the following message:

I'm going to be in Tokyo to give some lessons starting tomorrow afternoon. Would it be possible to meet before then?

They decided to meet at a hotel near Tokyo Station at eleven o'clock for tea. Hori said he had a previous appointment and wouldn't be able to go himself, but seemed to know what Eiko intended. "Be sure to listen carefully, you two," he said. "I'm pretty sure you'll learn something important."

Arriving with a wheeled carryall holding the gear for her lessons, Eiko seemed pleased to hear about Oba and Umemoto's progress and how they were feeling.

"Actually," Eiko said, "Tetsuya didn't want me to tell you this, but he asked me to meet with you today. He really wanted me to tell you something about myself that I shared with him two years ago. He sure looks out for his subordinates—such a gentleman!"

Oba and Umemoto looked at each other in shock.

What Eiko had told Hori two years ago was the story of how she ended up making a video that would get millions of views.

Eiko had started out as an aerobics instructor. Nevertheless, her body was less limber than most people and she couldn't do the splits at all. Aerobics didn't require doing the splits, but it was better to have a flexible body than not, and most of the people who were recognized as the best instructors could do beautiful splits.

At aerobics competitions, competitors would do high kicks and jumps, lifting their legs to the front and the sides. Muscle strength, muscle endurance, and flexibility were all called into question. Eiko never achieved very good results in individual competition.

Of course, scoring well at aerobics events and being a good instructor, although they seem related, are completely different things. Instructors who know how to teach and how to take care of and motivate their students remain more popular, and are more appreciated, than instructors who might be outstanding performers but tend to go their own way.

Eiko decided not to worry about her lack of flexibility. Still, not being able to even do the splits was something she couldn't talk about with anyone.

After Eiko had children, the world's interest had shifted from aerobics to yoga. The intense movements of aerobics had gotten harder as she had gotten older, too, so Eiko decided to switch to yoga, starting out as a student herself.

Yoga instruction was booming in Japan at the time but mainly focused on power yoga, a style completely different from what Eiko teaches now. Eager to gain a more flexible body, Eiko threw herself into yoga but soon lost her enthusiasm and nearly gave up.

In fact, she did quit for a time and even took other work. But this didn't last, either. She just didn't feel that she had found her place. Trying yoga one more time, she improved rapidly and soon found herself teaching. This time, though, she overdid it despite her inflexibility and ended up getting hurt, which brought things to a standstill and left her bogged down. She carried on despite the discomfort, holding things together with regular acupuncture and massage treatments, but soon realized that things were completely backward.

If her students were coming to Eiko to learn yoga because they wanted to be healthy and to enjoy themselves, what sense did it make for her to be unhealthy and unhappy herself?

What occurred to her then for the first time was the idea of a reasonable, effective stretching program for inflexible people. Nobody taught it to her, and she didn't copy anyone. She came up with a way to stretch for health and for fun that was both motivating and encouraging and resulted in the thrill and surprise of doing the splits.

The video she happened to shoot and post to the web spread virally through social media and was soon viewed a million times. If she had been limber from the start, she never would have had such a chance. It was precisely because she had been inflexible that she was able to develop an original method for doing the splits.

Both Oba and Umemoto listened intently to Eiko's story.

"Eiko," said Umemoto, "you struggled so much. I can't help seeing myself in your story."

"Tetsuya said almost the same thing two years ago," Eiko replied. "And also that the most important thing was to listen to what was in your heart and just keep doing it."

Oba was filled with a sense of gratitude for Hori's feelings, for Eiko's compassion, and for the opportunity to hear Eiko's story. In the end, no matter how far you go, it all comes down to you.

"There isn't actually all that much I can do as an instructor," said Eiko. "No matter how much encouragement I give, or how simply I arrange the method, in the end it comes down to the fact that some people follow through and some people don't."

Oba and Umemoto both nodded deeply.

"Ai," said Eiko, "I've never done much of the sort of work that you do, so all I can do for you is try to give you a sense, by moving your body, of the part of your brain that's wired to do what it sets out to do. Work and the splits and yoga and dieting are really all the same thing."

Eiko's "way of the splits" fell right into place for Umemoto, who had been worried about all sorts of things over the last few years. Stretching and the splits were more than just stretching and the splits; they were a means of "awakening" through the use of the body. Not waiting for instructions, or waiting for orders, but setting her own goals and moving forward of her own volition along a path that she believed in—*that* was a life all her own.

Oba and Umemoto fully understood what Hori had intended, and pledged to a beaming Eiko their commitment to achieving the splits.

PUSH FORWARD ON YOUR OWN PATH!

(Week 4 Explanation and Practice)

Monday evening arrived. Both Oba and Umemoto realized that they hadn't looked forward to a particular day so much since the school excursions and trips of their childhood.

"All right," said Hori, looking pleased, "just one more step to go!"

Oba and Umemoto didn't have the heart to tell Hori that they knew he had asked Eiko to meet with them. Remaining silent seemed like the best way to express their gratitude for what he had done.

"Did you learn something from talking with Eiko?" Hori asked. "When I was first learning to do the splits I couldn't help but see myself in her experience. Knowing the story behind the creation of the video, and realizing that I was asking for her help after seeing it, really moved me. After all, it was her awakening that was having such a positive effect on me, and now is having on the two of you. Only when you open up your own path instead of acting on the order of others are you able to come up with ideas for the kinds of things no one has done before. That's the message I hoped you two would get."

Both Oba and Umemoto wore expressions even brighter than before.

"Okay," Hori continued. "On to week four!"

Door Stretch

Finally, the last week! With the door stretch, since you let the walls take care of your legs, your goal of the splits should seem closer than ever. If you don't have a door to use, try the frog stretch.

BASIC STRETCHES TO DO EVERY DAY

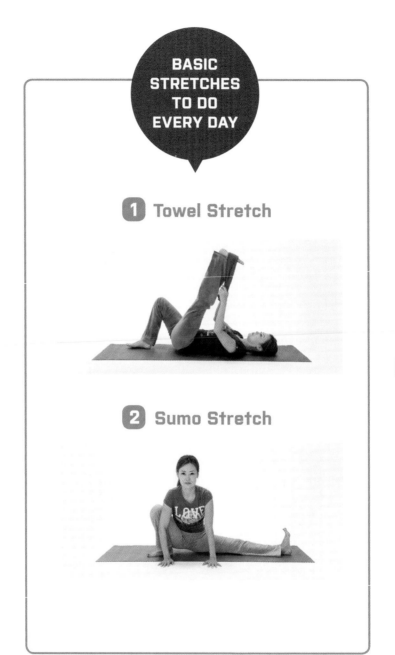

1 Towel Stretch

2 Sumo Stretch

+

3 Door Stretch

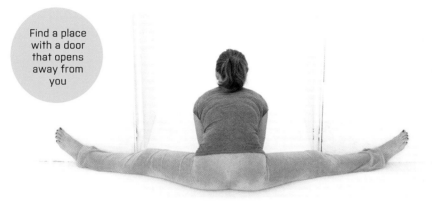

Find a place with a door that opens away from you

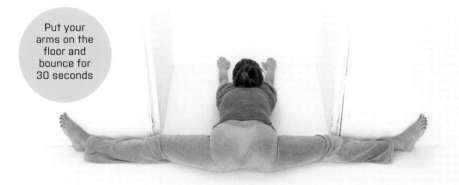

Put your arms on the floor and bounce for 30 seconds

1 Find a doorway whose walls on both sides are in the same plane and whose door opens away from you, then sit down in front of it with your legs spread.

2 Supporting your outstretched legs with the walls, lower your upper body forward and place your arms on the floor, stretching for 30 seconds while bouncing.

If you don't have a door:

FROG STRETCH

Spread your legs wide with your toes pointing out. Lower your hands to the floor and support your upper body, which will want to tumble forward, stretching for 30 seconds. If you cannot reach the floor with your hands, support your upper body by resting your elbows on your thighs near your knees.

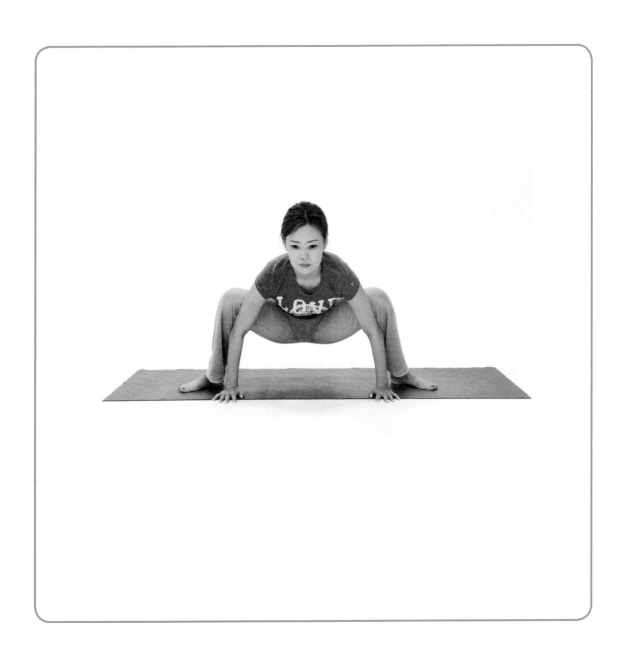

After four weeks, you're sure to see a change.

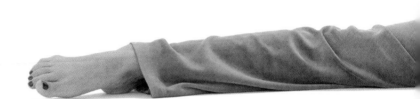

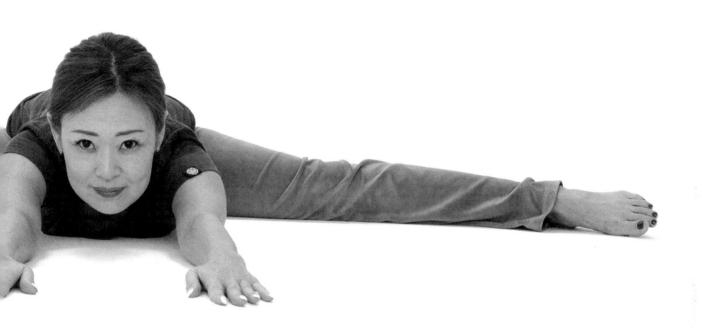

First, Umemoto tried the frog stretch. Although cautious at first, in the end she was able to smoothly touch the floor with her hands.

Next, all three of them opened the conference-room door and, after checking to see that there was no one in the hallway outside, tried the door stretch. Oba went first, and was able to spread his legs pretty wide and lean forward farther than he had expected.

"Okay, Makoto," said Hori. "I'm going to give you a little push."

Hori pushed Oba's back but the pressure didn't feel like much of a burden. He was really close to being able to do the splits. Then, just as Umemoto spread her legs to try the splits herself, they all heard a big group of people deep in serious conversation as they approached down the hallway. Someone was coming!

"Uh-oh," shouted Hori, "you two hide!" He hurriedly pushed the other two, dressed in their training wear, into the conference room, leapt in behind them, and shut the door with a bang. They made it just in time. "Whew!" he said. "That was close, you two. You just missed getting chewed out for being dressed like that at work."

"That's all right, Tetsuya," said Oba. "As long as you're here to share the scolding with us, I'm not worried."

"I think so, too," said Umemoto. "But, doesn't this feel like being one of the bad kids who hangs around school even after classes are out?"

"Who's being bad?" said Hori. "We're just following the path we believe in, so we ought to throw out our chests with confidence. Still, we are at the office, so I suppose we all ought to put our suits on first."

At Hori's words, all three of them burst into laughter.

FINALLY, THE TIME HAS COME

Finally, the day arrived.

It was Thursday, and Oba—his breathing somewhat measured as he tested his body—tried the splits that he had been aiming for. He spread his legs out wide, keeping his knees straight, exhaled with a "haa," and slowly lowered his upper body.

Ten centimeters to go. Then five.

No pain.

Then his elbows touched the floor.

He had done it!

"You did it!" shouted his wife, wide-eyed in surprise.

Oba thought it might have been the first time he had heard her shout like this since he confessed his feelings to her, back when they were students. In an oddly romantic pose with his chin in his hands, Oba felt slightly embarrassed.

"Dad," said Tsubasa, who had gotten out of bed when he heard the fuss. "That's awesome!" Oba had waited until he thought his son was asleep to try the splits, afraid that he would look ridiculous if he tried and failed.

The experience of having accomplished something with the support of his family, his boss, and his

143

colleague was even greater than he had imagined. He couldn't wait to show Hori, and wondered how Umemoto was doing.

Umemoto also achieved the splits late that same night. The moment she did, she felt so happy she thought her blood would boil and couldn't help letting out an audible whoop in her empty apartment.

She could tell that she had been more cheerful lately, not just on the surface but deep down. The night before, she had spoken with her mother on the telephone for the first time in a while. Her mother, of course, had no idea that Umemoto had been working on doing the splits every day. Umemoto had surprised herself by reacting in an unusually upbeat tone when her mother started in again on how she should be thinking about marriage.

If it was too late for love, then there was no need to do anything.

If she wanted romance, then she could pursue it.

If she didn't have time, she just needed to make time.

All she needed to do was go out to new places.

It didn't matter what others thought.

She just needed to follow her own path, of her own volition, in her own life.

That's all there was to it.

Umemoto remembered where she had been just a month before and felt rather proud of herself. On her white walls she imagined the faces of Director Hori, Eiko, and Makoto.

Doing the splits, with her elbows on the floor and her chin resting in the palms of her hands, she felt a mix of happiness, of hurting in a good way, and the fatigue of another long day that seemed to lull her into a state of suspension.

In a word, it felt really good. She was excited, yet felt on the verge of a deep sleep. This could be addictive. Maybe this was the "splits high" Eiko had talked about. For no particular reason, she started to cry.

The next morning when Oba and Umemoto ran into each other at work, they both immediately knew that the other had achieved the splits without even having to ask.

"So you did it, right?" said Umemoto.

"Yes," said Oba. "Yes, I did!"

"Me, too," said Umemoto, looking ready to jump for joy. "I can't wait to show Director Hori."

If there hadn't been anyone else around, Oba would probably have given her a hug. They decided to keep their success a secret from Hori until Monday evening.

Finally, the fateful end of the four weeks had arrived. Oba set picnic sheets down in the conference room and then showed off his splits first, followed by Umemoto. Hori nodded deeply again and again with tears in his eyes. When Umemoto stood up, Hori suddenly drew them both in by the shoulders.

"You've done so well," he said. "I knew this day would come. Congratulations!"

Umemoto was crying, too.

"You two can do anything now," Hori continued. "Whether at work or in your private lives, I want you to push straight on ahead in the direction you want to go."

Oba was all smiles.

"Now," said Hori, switching quickly into work mode, "I want the two of you to join a new project I'm going to direct myself. It's a big project that may decide the future of the company. We're going to start from scratch, developing new clients with the goal of stealing a thirty-percent share of the market. I want the two of you to start on the marketing."

This was a tall order, but when Oba and Umemoto instinctively looked at each other, the expressions of each were clear.

"We'll have regular meetings for the project here in this conference room at seven o'clock every Monday evening. Ai, go to General Affairs and have them block us in."

Oba and Umemoto lit up with smiles.

"And Makoto," said Hori, "I've got a new assignment for you: lose ten pounds. That shouldn't be any problem for you now. I want weekly reports!"

"Tetsuya, are you serious?"

"Ooh," said Umemoto. "I can't wait to see what Makoto looks like when he's trim."

The conference room exploded in laughter.

END

1   Keep your hips strong and flexible to function at your best. *Women's Nutrition Connection* 18, no. 9 (September 2015): 7. Food Science Source, EBSCOhost (accessed August 24, 2017).

2   Rubenstein LZ, Josephson KR. Falls and their prevention in elderly people: what does the evidence show? *Medical Clinics of North America* 2006, 90: 807–24.

3   Cascaes da Silva, et al. Effects of physical-exercise-based rehabilitation programs on the quality of life of patients with Parkinson's disease: A systematic review of randomized controlled trials. *Journal of Aging & Physical Activity* 24, no. 3 (July 2016): 484–96. *Social Sciences Abstracts* (H.W. Wilson), EBSCOhost (accessed August 24, 2017).

4   Hotta, Kazuki, et al. Stretching exercises enhance vascular endothelial function and improve peripheral circulation in patients with acute myocardial infarction. *International Heart Journal* 54, no. 2 (2013): 59–63. MEDLINE with Full Text, EBSCOhost (accessed August 24, 2017).

5   Enax, Laura, Eva Heiliger, Nadine Gier, and Bernd Weber. 2016. The influence of short-term aerobic exercise on food decision-making. Neuropsychoeconomics Conference Proceedings 43. Academic Search Complete, EBSCOhost (accessed August 23, 2017).

6   Alajmi, Nawal, et al. Appetite and energy intake responses to acute energy deficits in females versus males. *Medicine & Science in Sports & Exercise* 48, no. 3 (March 2016).

7   Jesudason, Rajiv, et al. Differential effects of static and cyclic stretching during elastase digestion on the mechanical properties of extracellular matrices. *Journal of Applied Physiology* 103, no. 3 (September 2007): 803–11. *SPORTDiscus with Full Text*, EBSCOhost (accessed August 25, 2017).

8   Jones, Donna. Bending the rules. *Sunday Telegraph* (Sydney) (n.d.): Business Source Corporate Plus, EBSCOhost (accessed August 24, 2017).

9   Behm, David George, et al. Acute bouts of upper and lower body static and dynamic stretching increase non-local joint range of motion. *European Journal of Applied Physiology* 116, no. 1 (January 2016): 241–49. MEDLINE with Full Text, EBSCOhost (accessed August 23, 2017).

10   http://www.stretchaflex.com/benefits-of-stretching#ixzz4qbMro8BM

11   Shellock FG and WE Prentice. 1985. Warming-up and stretching for improved physical performance and prevention of sports-related injuries. *Sports Medicine* 2, no. 4: 267–78. SPORTDiscus with Full Text, EBSCOhost (accessed August 25, 2017).

12   Bosu, Olatunde, et al. Stretching for prevention of exercise-related injury. *American Family Physician* 94, no. 7 (October 1, 2016): 547. MEDLINE with Full Text, EBSCOhost (accessed August 23, 2017).

13   Keep your hips strong and flexible to function at your best. 18, no. 9 (September 2015): 7. *Food Science Source*, EBSCOhost (accessed August 24, 2017).

14   Jones, Donna. Work your asana off. *Sunday Tasmanian* (Hobart)(n.d.): Business Source Corporate Plus, EBSCOhost (accessed August 24, 2017).

15   Inami, Takayuki, et al. 2015. Acute changes in peripheral vascular tonus and systemic circulation during static stretching. *Research in Sports Medicine* (Print) 23, no. 2: 167–78. MEDLINE with Full Text, EBSCOhost (accessed August 24, 2017).

16   Weider, Joe. It's no stretch. *Joe Weider's Muscle & Fitness* 69, no. 10 (October 2008): 30. SPORTDiscus with Full Text, EBSCOhost (accessed August 24, 2017).

EIKO

Eiko is a yoga instructor from Osaka who advocates "shake yoga," having begun teaching yoga after a decade working as an aerobics instructor. Her original "shake yoga" method has drawn attention as a fun, effective approach that can be enjoyed even by people who are inflexible or who suffer from lower-back pain. Having shown many people her techniques for achieving a more limber body in the course of teaching yoga, the video she released in 2015—"Stretches That Will Enable Even Inflexible People to Do the Splits"— went viral on Twitter and Facebook, reached millions of viewers on YouTube, and made her famous, as the Queen of Splits. Among her yoga students are those who can do the splits with ease even at the age of 70.

About the Author

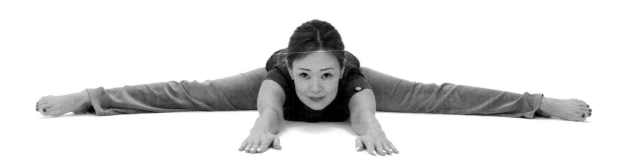

Underscored page references indicate sidebars. **Boldface** references indicate photographs.